Hajar Abedi
Clara Magnier
Kavini Rabel
Arunav Munjal
Divya Kamath
Kashish Grover
Shenbei Fan
Shyan Mascarenhas
Plinio P. Morita
Jennifer Boger
Alexander Wong
George Shaker

A Comprehensive Review of Gait

Exploring Existing Technologies, Methods, and Analyses

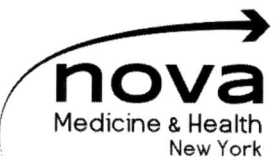

Copyright © 2025 by Nova Science Publishers, Inc.
DOI: https://doi.org/10.52305/OELL2084

All rights reserved. No part of this book may be reproduced, stored in a retrieval system or transmitted in any form or by any means: electronic, electrostatic, magnetic, tape, mechanical photocopying, recording or otherwise without the written permission of the Publisher.

We have partnered with Copyright Clearance Center to make it easy for you to obtain permissions to reuse content from this publication. Simply navigate to this publication's page on Nova's website and locate the "Get Permission" button below the title description. This button is linked directly to the title's permission page on copyright.com. Alternatively, you can visit copyright.com and search by title, ISBN, or ISSN.

For further questions about using the service on copyright.com, please contact:
Copyright Clearance Center
Phone: +1-(978) 750-8400   Fax: +1-(978) 750-4470   E-mail: info@copyright.com

NOTICE TO THE READER

The Publisher has taken reasonable care in the preparation of this book, but makes no expressed or implied warranty of any kind and assumes no responsibility for any errors or omissions. No liability is assumed for incidental or consequential damages in connection with or arising out of information contained in this book. The Publisher shall not be liable for any special, consequential, or exemplary damages resulting, in whole or in part, from the readers' use of, or reliance upon, this material. Any parts of this book based on government reports are so indicated and copyright is claimed for those parts to the extent applicable to compilations of such works.

Independent verification should be sought for any data, advice or recommendations contained in this book. In addition, no responsibility is assumed by the Publisher for any injury and/or damage to persons or property arising from any methods, products, instructions, ideas or otherwise contained in this publication.

The Publisher assumes no responsibility for any statements of fact or opinion expressed in the published contents.

This publication is designed to provide accurate and authoritative information with regard to the subject matter covered herein. It is sold with the clear understanding that the Publisher is not engaged in rendering legal or any other professional services. If legal or any other expert assistance is required, the services of a competent person should be sought. FROM A DECLARATION OF PARTICIPANTS JOINTLY ADOPTED BY A COMMITTEE OF THE AMERICAN BAR ASSOCIATION AND A COMMITTEE OF PUBLISHERS.

Additional color graphics may be available in the e-book version of this book.

Library of Congress Cataloging-in-Publication Data

ISBN: 979-8-89530-470-9 (Softcover)
ISBN: 979-8-89530-530-0 (eBook)

Published by Nova Science Publishers, Inc. † New York

To the researchers and innovators dedicated to advancing gait analysis and improving lives - may this work contribute to the progress of science and healthcare.
And to those who walk the path of discovery, may every step bring you closer to knowledge and impact.

Contents

List of Tables		vii
List of Figures		ix
Preface		xi
Chapter 1	Introduction	1
Chapter 2	Background on Gait Analysis	3
Chapter 3	Technologies Available for Gait Analysis	11

    3.1. Non-Contact Devices 11
        3.1.1. Pressure Mats and Walkways 11
        3.1.2. Motion Capture 15
        3.1.3. Force Plates 17
        3.1.4. Infrared Thermal Cameras 18
    3.2. Radar Systems 19
        3.2.1. Continuous Wave (CW) 20
        3.2.2. Frequency Modulated Continuous Wave (FMCW) 21
        3.2.3. Impulse-Radio Ultra-Wide Band (IR-UWB) 24
        3.2.4. Pulse-Doppler Ultra-Wide Band (UWB) 25
    3.3. Contact Devices for Gait Analysis 28
        3.3.1. Wearables and Inertial Measurements Units (IMU) Sensors 28
        3.3.2. Gait Analyses through Footwear and Insoles 39
        3.3.3. Stride Analyzers 42

Chapter 4	**Pathological Implications of Gait**	**45**
	4.1. General Predictions from Gait	45
	4.2. Gait Analysis for Decline of Cognitive Function and Dementia	51
	4.3. Gait Analysis and Central Nervous System	62
	4.4. Gait Analysis and Fall Prediction	70
	4.5. Gait Analysis and Mortality	77
	4.6. Gait Analysis and Cardiovascular Risk	82
	4.7. Gait Analysis and Stroke	85
	4.8. Gait Analysis and Neurological Pathology	88
Chapter 5	**Discussion and Conclusion**	**91**
References		**97**
Index		**115**

List of Tables

Table 2.1. Operational definitions of gait parameters 5
Table 2.2. Significant change in gait variability parameters 5
Table 2.3. Quantitative reference values (mean and standard deviation) for spatiotemporal gait parameters 6
Table 2.4. Assessment of gait parameters 7
Table 3.1. Types of radar systems 26
Table 3.2. Contact devices for gait analysis 39
Table 4.1. Gait and general predictions 49
Table 4.2. Gait analysis for decline of cognitive function and dementia 58
Table 4.3. Gait analysis and central nervous system 67
Table 4.4. Gait analysis and fall prediction 74
Table 4.5. Gait analysis and mortality 80
Table 4.6. Results of the survival after one year according to the baseline speed 82
Table 4.7. Gait analysis and cardiovascular risk 84
Table 4.8. Gait analysis and stroke 87
Table 5.1. Summary of the methods used and the pathologies assessed 95

List of Figures

Figure 2.1. Gait cycle consisting of parameters during stance and swing phase. 3
Figure 3.1. GAITRite®. 12
Figure 3.2. Stepscan® System, a pressure-sensitive electronic floor tile device. 13
Figure 3.3. Zebris FDM-T. 14
Figure 3.4. "Valkyrie" camera. 16
Figure 3.5. "Vero" Vicon system. 16
Figure 3.6. Microsoft Kinect v2. 16
Figure 3.7. AX3 sensor. 33
Figure 3.8. Shimmer 3. 35
Figure 3.9. CV4 sensor. 36
Figure 3.10. V4 sensor. 36
Figure 3.11. RunScribe devices. 41
Figure 3.12. OpenGo insoles 42

Preface

Gait, the simple act of walking, is a fundamental yet complex movement that reflects an individual's overall health and well-being. In recent years, advancements in technology have significantly enhanced our ability to analyze gait patterns, leading to new insights in fields such as healthcare, rehabilitation, neurology, and artificial intelligence-driven movement assessment. This monograph aims to provide a thorough explanation of current gait analysis methodologies, emerging technologies, and their implications in various domains.

The motivation behind this work stems from the growing need for accurate, non-invasive, and reliable gait assessment techniques that can improve diagnosis, treatment, and overall patient care. From traditional motion capture systems to advanced radar-based methods, the ability to monitor and interpret human gait has evolved considerably. By compiling state-of-the-art research and practical applications, this book serves as a valuable resource for researchers, clinicians, engineers, and students who seek to understand and contribute to the field of gait analysis.

The monograph is structured into three main sections. The first section provides an overview of gait analysis, including fundamental concepts and historical developments. The second section delves into the diverse technologies available for gait assessment, ranging from wearable sensors to radar-based systems. The final section explores the pathological implications of gait, examining its role in detecting neurodegenerative diseases, fall risk, cardiovascular conditions, and more.

This work would not have been possible without the contributions of esteemed colleagues and collaborators who have shared their expertise and insights. I extend my deepest gratitude to all those who have supported this endeavor, including my co-authors, mentors, and the scientific community whose research continues to inspire innovation in this field.

It is my hope that this monograph will serve as a comprehensive reference for those seeking to advance gait analysis and its applications. Whether you are a researcher investigating new methodologies, a clinician looking to integrate gait analysis into medical practice, or a student eager to explore the complexities of human movement, I trust that this book will provide valuable knowledge and inspiration.

Hajar Abedi
February 2025

Chapter 1

Introduction

"Put one foot in front of the other." The manner of walking consisting of the continuous lifting and setting down of each foot can be defined as gait [1]. Gait is progressively being considered one of the most important daily activities while also acting as an indicator for long-term and acute health status changes, such as the detection of fall risks [2]. The instinctive character of this pattern could be an opportunity to analyze, detect, and even predict changes in health and cognition [3]. Parameters for gait can be utilized as attainable clinical markers to determine the risk of functional decline for neurological pathologies such as Alzheimer's and dementia without invasive detection systems [4]. Beyond neurological pathology, gait can be related to cardiovascular disease due to its involvement during physical effort [5]. Numerous technological devices are being developed to extract beneficial data from individual gait patterns. These existing technologies can be used to detect changes in people's gait patterns, especially in older adults. This information could be used to further support the detection and analysis of parameters related to changes in mobility, cognition, and frailty. This monograph aims to provide a thorough exploration of gait assessment methodologies, emerging technologies, and their real-world applications. The book is structured into several key sections:

- The first section introduces the fundamental principles of gait analysis, covering the biomechanics of movement, key gait parameters, and historical developments in the field.
- The second section delves into various technological advancements, from motion capture systems and wearable sensors to radar-based monitoring and machine learning-driven gait classification.
- The third section explores clinical applications, discussing the role of gait assessment in neurology, rehabilitation, cardiovascular health, and aging-related mobility impairments.

This book is intended for researchers, biomedical engineers, clinicians, and students seeking a comprehensive understanding of gait analysis. It bridges the gap between fundamental gait concepts and state-of-the-art technologies, offering insights into both theoretical foundations and practical applications. By the end of this monograph, readers will gain a deep appreciation of the complexities of human gait, its significance in health monitoring, and the future directions of gait research and technology.

Chapter 2
Background on Gait Analysis

"Gait analysis is the systematic study of human locomotion" [6]. Gait analysis focuses on the technical side of gait assessment, which looks to make gait measurements using available technologies to measure features such as walking speed and joint angles [7]. Gait analysis measurements can be made using technologies such as electromyography (EMG) recordings that provide users with visual presentations of gait. This builds up the movements of walking or the gait cycle, which can be used for physical examinations [1].

The most basic description of the gait is the gait cycle [1]. It is composed of two phases: the stance phase (when the foot remains in contact with the ground) and the swing phase (when the foot is not in contact with the ground). Each phase can be decomposed into different subparts, such as the initial heel strike or the terminal swing, as shown in Figure 2.1 [8].

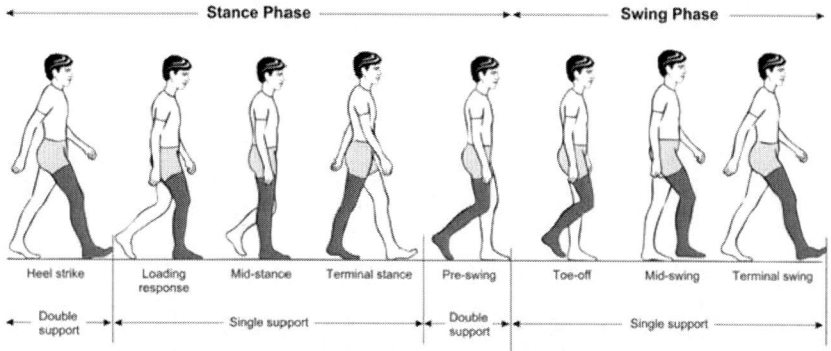

Figure 2.1. Gait cycle consisting of parameters during stance and swing phase [8].

There are multiple gait parameters (e.g., gait speed, swing phase time, stance phase time, swing phase variability, stance phase variability, cadence, etc.). Some parameters are derived from others or have been shown to be highly correlated. For example, mediolateral trunk acceleration and step width seem to have a quadratic relation to gait speed [9]. A factor analysis of multiple spatiotemporal gait parameters conducted in [10] reported a complete vision of existing parameters, and reference values have been added to a normative database of gait parameters for healthy individuals. The values were obtained with the electronic walkway GAITRite® [11]. Table 2.1 defines several of the parameters studied, which were classified into different domains: rhythm, phase, variability, pace, and base of support.

A study using a 24 GHz micro-Doppler radar has proven a statistically significant difference in the leg motion parameters in both the stance and swing phases for healthy individuals and those affected by gait disorders [12]. Researchers extracted the following parameters: mean walking velocity, maximum walking velocity, mean leg velocity in the swing phase, degree of variation of leg velocity in the swing phase, mean leg velocity in the stance phase, and degree of variation of leg velocity in the stance phase. Studying the leg motion parameters is relevant because they reflect the deterioration of balance ability due to aging and cannot be controlled by the subject's will.

When using gait speed as a predictor of disease, it is beneficial to know if gait speed declines only with age. A study on the Baltimore Longitudinal Study of Aging has analyzed the walking parameters of 362 participants aged 60 to 89 with a mean follow-up time of 3.2 years [13]. Age was not associated with the decline of gait speed when controlling for gait and demographic characteristics. A 3-dimensional motion capture system and a force capture system have been used to evaluate the walking parameters (gait speed during a 6-meter walk, cadence, stride length, percent of a gait cycle in double stance, anterior-posterior mechanical work expenditure, and medial-lateral work expenditure). On the contrary, Viccaro et al. have analyzed the walking speed of 358 healthy people using accelerometry and an algorithm to transform the data and demonstrated a decrease in walking speed of -0.0037 m/s per year [14]. There is an association between walking speed and age in free living. However, this result is not the difference in walking speed of the same individual at two different times; it is the comparison of the walking speed of various age participants. Hence, we cannot exclude the possibility that all the slower participants had a slow gait speed that can be a predictor of future pathology.

Moreover, a study published in 2010 defined the meaningful changes in gait variability in older adults [15]. Researchers collected data from 1,148 participants in the Einstein Aging Study with a 12-foot (3.7-meter) instrumented walkway on which participants had to walk at their usual speed. They defined gait variability as "the within-subject standard deviation derived from all the right steps recorded over two trials." Table 2.2 summarizes the results of the study. The significant change in gait speed and step width was also assessed, but the results were not good enough to conclude a value.

Background on Gait Analysis

Table 2.1. Operational definitions of gait parameters

Spatiotemporal parameters	
Gait speed (m/s)	The distance walked divided by the walking time
Spatial parameters	
Step length (cm)	The length measured parallel to the Line of Progression of the body, from the contact of the heel from the previous footfall to the contact of the heel from the opposing footfall. It can be calculated as the covered distance divided by the number of completed steps.
Step width (cm)	The distance measured between lines of progression of the right and left foot. Mediolateral distance between the heels in the double support phase.
Stride length (cm)	The distance measured parallel to the Line of Progression, between the heel points the same foot for two consecutive footprints.
Temporal parameters	
Cadence (steps/minutes)	The number of steps by minutes.
Step time (s)	The time between the initial contact of one foot and the initial contact of the opposite foot.
Stride time (s)	The time between two initial contacts of the same foot (two consecutive footfalls).
Stance time (s)	The duration between the initial contact and final contact of the same foot.
Swing time (s)	The duration between the last contact of a footfall and the initial contact of the following footfall
Single support time (s)	The duration of the swing phase where only one limb is in contact with the ground.
Double support time (s)	The duration of the phase of support on both feet.

Table 2.2. Significant change in gait variability parameters

Parameters	Stance time	Swing time	Step length
Significant variability	0.01 s	0.01 s	0.25 cm

The reliability of step-to-step variability for patients with neurodegenerative pathologies and healthy participants has been investigated in a 2018 study [16]. Researchers used GAITRite® to analyze the gait parameters at slow, normal, and fast speeds for 29 patients with different intermediary types of Parkinson's disease and 25 healthy individuals. They concluded that errors in gait speed analysis were minimized when the gait variability was based on 40 steps and that step width was the most reliable parameter for all groups and speeds. However, variability at a slow speed is not reliable for Parkinson's disease patients. To conclude, studying gait variability for Parkinson's disease patients is reliable at usual and fast speeds and best at 40 steps.

A complete analysis led by two consortiums (Biomathics and the Canadian Gait Consortium) published in 2017 provides consensus guidance for clinical and spatiotemporal gait analysis and reference values for spatiotemporal gait analysis [17]. Researchers used two different databases, "Gait Cognition and Decline" (GOOD) and Generation 100 (Gen100), that had gait assessments with GAITRite® for individuals older than 65 years. The guidance for clinical gait analysis was defined with either a minimal or complete data set. The minimal data set should be composed of four gait parameters (walking speed, value, and variation of stride time, swing time, and stride width) evaluated in normal walking conditions. The parameters added for the full dataset are the value and variation of stride length, stance time, single and double support, and stride time velocity. All the parameters should be measured at standard walking speed, maximum walking speed, and two dual-task conditions (one by counting backward from fifty and one by enumerating animal names). For both minimum and full datasets, a minimum of 400 steps and three consecutive gait cycles for both the left and right sides should be assessed. Researchers suggested that all adults older than 65 be examined yearly for gait disorders, and everyone with a history of falls or acute treatment should also be examined. The values of the mean and the standard deviation for the total population data are reported in Table 2.3.

Table 2.3. Quantitative reference values (mean and standard deviation) for spatiotemporal gait parameters

Mean values of parameters ± standard deviation	Total population (n = 954)
Mean Age (years) ± SD	72.8 ± 4.8
Mean Stride time (ms) ± SD	1123.7 ± 122.4
Mean swing time (ms) ± SD	414.1 ± 40.2
Mean stance time (ms) ± SD	706.6 ± 91.2
Mean single support time (ms) ± SD	414.3 ± 39.8
Mean double support time (ms) ± SD	292.6 ± 71.0
Mean stride length (cm) ± SD	134.1 ± 18.9
Mean stride width (cm) ± SD	9.9 ± 3.1
Mean walking speed (cm/s) ± SD	121.5 ± 23.4
Mean stride velocity ± SD	119.9 ± 22.5

Several publications analyzed the timed up-and-go (TUG) in addition to gait speed when assessing an association between parameters and a particular pathology. TUG is an evaluation of physical form during which the patient must rise from a chair, walk a few meters back, and sit down on the chair.

Table 2.4. Assessment of gait parameters

Study	Sample	Method of Analysis	Parameters analyzed	Conclusion about parameters
Gait variability and the risk of incident mobility disability in community-dwelling older adults [19] (2007)	379 adults (mean age = 79 years)	Computerized walkway	Gait speed, step length, stance time and stance time variability	Only stance time variability is a predictor of disability
Gait variability and fall risk in community-living older adults: a 1-year prospective study [20] (2001)	52 community-living aged 70 and older	Walk of six minutes wearing force-sensitive insoles	Gait rhythm, the timing of gait speed, stride time, swing time, stride and swing time variability	Only stride time variability could predict falls
Decline in gait performance detected by an electronic walkway system in 907 older adults of the population-based KORA-Age study [21] (2013)	907 adults aged between 65 and 91 years	Electronic walkway GAITRite®	Different walking speeds, dual-task walking, the impact of endoprostheses and mobility aids	Fast speed, dual-task walking, age-related endoprostheses and mobility can predict a decline of gait performance
The reliability of gait variability measures for individuals with Parkinson's disease and healthy older adults – The effect of gait speed [16] (2018)	29 Parkinson's disease patient and 25 healthy participants aged over 65 years	Electronic walkway GAITRite®	Gait variability	Gait variability is reliable at a usual and fast rhythm to analyze Parkinson's disease patients and 40 steps are the most reliable distance of analysis
Functional assessment in older adults: Should we use timed up and go or gait speed test? [18] (2014)	37 frail participants	Motion capture-system	Timed up and go and gait speed	Gait speed is more representative of the motor ability than the timed up and go
Is timed up and go better than gait speed in predicting health, function, and falls in older adults? [14] (2011)	457 adults aged 65 years and older	Stopwatch (4 meters)	Timed up and go and gait speed	Gait speed and TUG are both good predictors of outcomes

Table 2.4. (Continued)

Study	Sample	Method of Analysis	Parameters analyzed	Conclusion about parameters
Guidelines for assessment of gait and reference values for spatiotemporal gait parameters in older adults: The biomathics and Canadian gait consortiums initiative [17] (2017)	2 different databases	GAITRite® system	/	The minimum dataset to assessed gait disorders should be walking speed, value, and derivation of stride time, stand time and stride width at a usual speed. Gait should be assessed every year after 65 years old

The most representative test between TUG and gait speed for 37 frail patients was investigated by Kubicki [18]. Gait speed and TUG were assessed with an active motion-capture system. Different pairs of variables were plotted to calculate the corresponding Pearson correlation coefficients (PCC[1]). The conclusion was that gait speed was more representative of the motor ability of frail patients than the TUG. Another study with a larger sample evaluated whether TUG was a better predictor of poor outcomes than gait speed [14]. Thus, researchers have assessed the baseline gait speed and TUG of 457 adults aged older than 65 years with a stopwatch. They also used different tests (Baseline Gait speed and TUG) to measure health decline and outcomes with a 1-year follow-up. They concluded that gait speed and TUG were both good predictors of outcomes; therefore, adding a TUG test to a gait speed test might not be useful.

Gait analysis is used in different fields [7] (e.g., sports analysis, clinical assessment, and human recognition). Gait is a reliable factor that is easy to measure and can predict a decline in cognitive function, neurodegenerative diseases, falls, cardiovascular diseases, and stroke, as will be explained in this monograph. This literary review aims to describe what has already been done to study walking gait and what we know about the association between walking and health. It will first report the different analysis methods and then describe the association that has been proven between gait parameters and various pathologies.

---

[1] Pearson correlation coefficients (PCC) depict a linear relationship, with values ranging closer to negative -1 being a negative relationship, while values closer to positive 1 are a positive relationship.

Chapter 3
Technologies Available for Gait Analysis

Different technologies are used to analyze gait and predict pathologies. This chapter aims to describe existing methods and examine their reliability. Here, commonly used devices will be covered, providing a background on the features of each device and how they have been utilized concerning gait analysis. The introduced devices are of ranging accessibility to provide insight into alternative technologies that can either be used at home without clinical supervision or those of higher accuracy only found in clinical setting environments on account of cost and expertise. This chapter separates these devices and technologies into two distinct categories: non-contact devices and contact devices.

3.1. Non-Contact Devices

In this monograph, non-contact devices are classified as devices that do not involve body contact with individuals and are used as an alternative form of data collection for gait analysis. These devices monitor and record gait parameters without requiring physical attachment to participants. These devices can be more convenient, as less setup is required when connecting the device to the individual. This chapter aims to disclose several available non-contact devices used to monitor gait, which could be classified into five categories: Pressure Mats and Walkways, Motion Capture Devices, Force Plates, Infrared Thermal Cameras, and Radar.

3.1.1. Pressure Mats and Walkways

The GAITRite® system is a portable electronic walkway with embedded pressure sensors to measure gait patterns in time and space with an automated acquisition (Table 1) [11]. This pressure mat has a smooth top surface, allowing the mat to lie flat on the ground with the ability to be rolled up so that the set-up takes minimal time. GAITRite® offers multiple walkways for specific intended uses, either for research or clinical purposes [11]. The GAITRite® mat functions as a footfall that activates the sensors and deactivates with the toe-off; thus, a recording of consecutive footfalls in time is obtained. Electronically inactive extensions can be attached at each end of the walkway so that initial acceleration and final deceleration are not recorded [11].

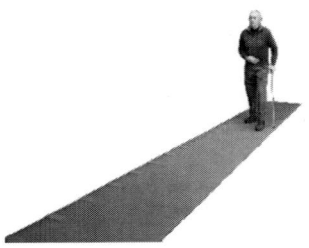

Figure 3.1. GAITRite® [11].

Researchers and clinicians who use the GAITRite® system can directly obtain information about gait parameters, including gait speed, cadence, and gait variability. Its accuracy for the spatial and temporal parameters of gait was investigated in several studies, one example being [22]. This research assessed the validity and reliability of the mat compared to the paper-and-pencil method for spatial measures and video-based methods for temporal measures, while the following parameters were studied: cadence, walking speed, stride lengths, right and left steps, and step times. The GAITRite® system was demonstrated to be a valid and reliable method of gait assessment. However, GAITRite® costs around 27 995 USD for a mat with a 4.27-meter (14-foot) detection zone and 16 128 sensors. This pricing can pose an issue for the development of good gait analysis on a regular basis, given that attending physicians might not be able to afford one for their office. The GAITRite® Walkway is used as the gold standard for gait analysis and is referred to multiple times throughout this paper as a comparison for the other devices mentioned.

Stepscan®, as shown in Figure 3.2, has also developed a multi-tile pressure-sensitive mat named Stepscan® Pedway which can be used for gait analysis [23]. Three different configurations exist: the 2' x 8' walkway, the 6' x 4' L-shaped walkway, and the 4' x 4' square platform. It has a 5-millimeter sensor resolution, and the sensor density is 4 sensors/cm².

Technologies Available for Gait Analysis 13

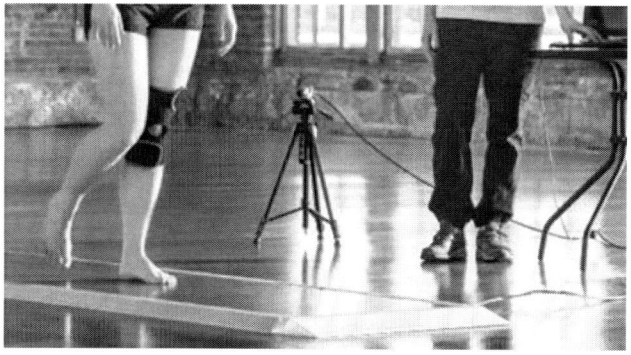

Figure 3.2. Stepscan® System, a pressure-sensitive electronic floor tile device [23].

The Stepscan® Pedway has been used in a previous study to acquire participants' spatial and temporal gait parameters [24]. The Stepscan® software provided mean data as it produced summary data and not data from individual gait cycles. Based on the limitations listed by Walford et al. [24], the Stepscan® Pedway was inadequate for obtaining abnormal gait pattern data.

Other pressure mats exist for gait analysis, such as the Zeno Walkway from Protokinetics [25]. This pressure mat can analyze spatiotemporal parameters of gait, the center of pressure trajectories, and relative pressures. When compared against the GAITRite® Walkway, the validity of the Zeno Walkway was found to be moderate to excellent for spatiotemporal parameters when used for older adults [26].

Another method used for gait assessment is using optical sensors such as the OptoGait system from MicroGate [27]. The system is composed of a transmitting and a receiving bar containing 96 LEDs that communicate with the corresponding opposite bar at an infrared frequency. The two bars are to be stationed on the floor, and the participant's movements when walking between the bars cause interruptions of communication, which are interpreted to find the position and the duration of the movement [27]. The system can be used on a treadmill in order to collect standard gait cycle data [28]. OptoGait has created supporting software to make information about gait (or other activities) easily accessible. The OptoGait software is organized into three sections: patient data, tests, and results [28]. This system costs roughly 2800 USD, and a minimum of 3-meter length is recommended for gait analysis. A 2014 publication [29] explained how the OptoGait system works and offered a protocol. An example of a representative report that can be obtained with the software demonstrated that step length, stride length, stance phase, swing phase, single support, load response, pre-swing, step time, gait cycle, cadence, and speed could be obtained with the software [29]. Also, the validity of the system has been investigated in [30]. For this study, the accuracy of OptoGait was measured compared to the GAITRite® system for an 8.4-meter distance. Values were compared for cycle time, stance time, swing time, step length, cadence, and walking speed. The statistical analysis used the intraclass correlation coefficient (ICC)[2], the 95% limits of agreement (LOA)[3], the bias, and the standard error of the estimate [29]. The ICC values were between 0.933 and 0.999, which means that OptoGait is a valid system. However, the cycle and stance time were always significantly longer for OptoGait, and the swing time, step length, cadence, and walking speed were significantly lower, meaning that the GAITRite® system and the OptoGait system cannot be interchanged [30].

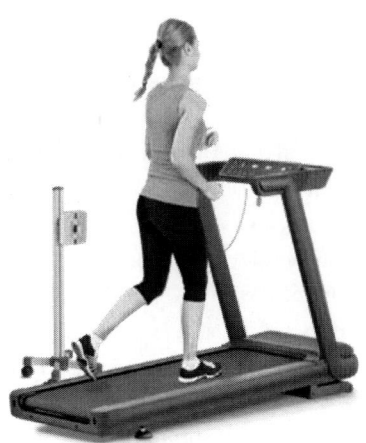

Figure 3.3. Zebris FDM-T [31].

Zebris has developed different frequency division multiplexing (FDM) systems for gait and posture analysis (Figure 3.3) [31]. The FDM systems are pressure platforms with embedded capacitive pressure sensors on which participant software and EMG data are used to complete gait analysis with a muscle analysis. All platforms' width and height are 0.4 meters and 2.1

---

[2] A statistic that is used to describe quantities based on a standard unit that are usually grouped together. Acceptable values for ICC range from around 0.75 to 0.90.
[3] A method that is used to compare two different methods of measurement by finding the mean difference.

centimeters respectively, while their lengths vary between 0.5 meters and 3 meters. Also, platforms larger than 1.5 meters can be combined with another platform of the same size to increase the sensor area. Zebris has also commercialized the FDM-T System, which is a treadmill ergometer with an embedded matrix of capacitive force sensors [31]. The treadmill's movement is compensated so that a stable gait analysis or running analysis can be realized. The patient's gait can be analyzed with and without shoes, and hence the influence of the shoes on the quality of gait can be investigated. Moreover, the software created for the pressure platform can provide a virtual environment for gait to force the participant to have constant variation in their walking and balancing modes. Another treadmill offered by Zebris is the Rehawalk®, which is designed to analyze and treat disorders [32]. The system includes a large monitor mounted in front of a treadmill, a processing unit, and virtual feedback training. The participant is maintained on the platform with a harness. The validity of this treadmill was assessed and it was found to have excellent reliability for temporal parameters with a displayed ICC value of ≥ 0.9 [33]. The study also determined that the device was easy to use, given its setup.

3.1.2. Motion Capture

Motion capture can be used for gait analysis using motion analysis technologies. They can quantify individual body segments in two- or three-dimensional space, which is often required for gait analysis. This method allows for precise measurements to be made, even when given complex movements that meet the specific needs of its intended purposes [34]. Motion capture is the recording of 2D or 3D movements with the use of one or several cameras. Initially, standard cameras were used; the participants had markers on their bodies, and complimentary motion capture software was used to process the data. Now, infrared cameras can also be used with reflective markers. The Vicon brand developed several cameras that can be used for gait analysis, with two examples shown in Figure 3.4 and Figure 3.5 [35]. The Vicon Nexus software can then be used to process the raw data. A Vicon product was used in a 2013 study [36]. The study aimed to compare the gait parameters of three categories of participants. For this purpose, a 6-camera Vicon 612 system was used to measure thirty-one 14-millimeter markers, and the following parameters were obtained and compared: gait speed, stride length, stride width, stance phase of the gait cycle, and stride time. In 2016, the Vicon MX (Vicon), a 3D motion capture system, was also used with 55 reflective markers for gait analysis [37]. The gait speed, step length, step width, stance time, swing time, and step frequency of 191 adults were measured using this system.

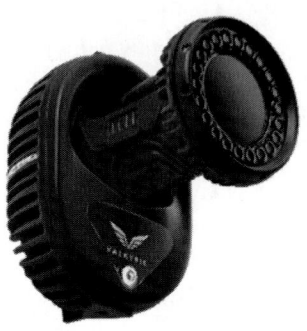

Figure 3.4. "Valkyrie" camera [35].

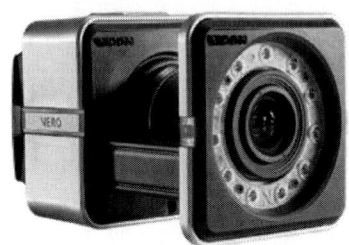

Figure 3.5. "Vero" Vicon system [35].

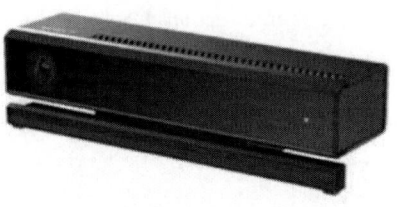

Figure 3.6. Microsoft Kinect v2 [38].

Another commercialized camera is the Kinect v2 from Microsoft, as shown in Figure 3.6 [38]. It can extract data from 3D skeletal modelling and has a camera with a colour (1920 x 1080 pixels) and depth (512 x 424 pixels), higher than the first version. Its validity and accuracy were assessed in a 2017 study [39]. The reference system was an infrared camera, and the calculated parameters were the step length, the step width, the step time, the stride time, and the foot swing velocity. Through this comparison, the study determined that the Kinect v2 met the standard for performing an effective clinical assessment. The device was determined to have excellent capacity to measure spatiotemporal measurements for step length and width [39].

RGB-D (Red Green Blue-Depth) cameras are a type of depth-sensing device associated with an RGB camera [40]. The classical image from an RGB camera is increased with depth information on a pixel basis. It can be used for human motion analysis or gait analysis, as done by Fosty et al. [41]. RGB-D cameras cannot directly be used to analyze gait, especially for older adults, since they pose limitations when obtaining intensive physical activity data with minimal data collection from the lower limbs. The development of a Point Cloud-Based System (PCBS) has allowed researchers to increase the representation of physical activity [41]. The measurements were realized with a standard treadmill on 36 participants; only the walking speed was calculated, and it was demonstrated to be accurate and reliable with a bias of 0.013 ms and $0.63 < ICC < 0.91$. However, this system requires a treadmill for the PCBS and the RGB-D camera, which can pose limitations given the difficulty of use.

3.1.3. Force Plates

Force plates make use of piezoelectric[4] measurement technology to register forces and movements for gait analysis. Parameters such as the impulse response, the frequency, and the frequency range can be changed. The Kistler brand [42] has created a series of force plates that can be used in different contexts, for example, swimming or jumping. Several plates can be put together to create a mat for the measurement. Some plates are also portable; however, the weight of the plates is greater than 5 kg. The non-portable plates weigh between 17.5 kg and 80 kg. The data obtained from the Kistler force plates can be processed using MARS software. Thus, information about balance and stability can be obtained by analyzing the shifts in the center of

---

[4] The ability to produce an electric charge resulting from applied mechanical stress.

pressure. The Kistler brand force plate was verified in a study to calibrate force sensors. The accuracy of the force plate was tested as a reference for calibration by applying varying weight loading methods to the force plate [43].

Another brand, AMTI, developed force plates for gait analysis [44]. Different models are available, such as the AccuGait Optimized™, a 502 x 502-millimeter force plate weighing 11 kg, and hence, several of them are needed for a gait analysis. It can be used with the corresponding NetForce software for data acquisition and the BioAnalysis software to obtain information concerning gait, balance, and power. Parameters of gait, such as stance time, velocity, the center of pressure, or maximum and minimum power, are outcomes of the software.

The influence of targeting on force plates has been investigated by Verniba et al. [45]. Participants were asked to walk on a treadmill with an embedded force plate. First, experiments were performed without targeting, and then targeting experiments, where participants had to walk within the bounds of a tape outline located on the last force plate, were performed. The spatiotemporal parameters calculated were walking speed, step time, and double support time. The results showed no significant difference for spatiotemporal parameters with or without targeting. Moreover, a Kistler brand force plate was used to determine the stride length, stride duration, single support, double support, swing duration, and periods of the gait cycle of 18 participants with a force plate. The platform was a Kistler 900 x 600-millimeter and a Kistler eight-channel charge amplifier. Force plates are very useful for the analysis of balance and posture. Still, they are not the most precise and accurate solution for gait analysis because not all the spatiotemporal parameters can be obtained with force plates. Furthermore, the AMTI or Kistler force plates must be calibrated by technicians with specific training, making the devices less accessible.

3.1.4. Infrared Thermal Cameras

Infrared thermal cameras have been used to create gait estimations through measurements of the participant's body temperature [46]. Thermal technology accurately functions as the body's skin emissivity[5] is 0.98 ± 0.01. This variable

---

[5] The ability of a surface to emit energy as thermal energy, expressed as a ratio.

is separate from the emissivity of the skin's other variables, such as pigmentation[6], absorptivity, reflectivity[7], and transmissivity[8].

An infrared thermal camera was compared to GAITRite® as a walking speed measurement technology in a study. The study concluded that thermal systems could be used efficiently for gait analysis as this technology was proven successful in identifying walking speeds used for indicating frailty [46]. The study utilizing thermal-based technologies as a more practical approach for collecting image gait recognition [47]. They reported that the study achieved over 80% in gait recognition using the modified link model and support vector machine method[9] [48]. The Chinese Academy of Sciences (CASIA) has created two databases known as the CASIA B and C databases [49]. The CASIA C database is one of the first databases to include data from a thermal infrared spectrum (besides the visual spectrum). The use of this technology allows for gait recognition information in nighttime settings [49]. CASIA-C collected data from participants' walking conditions (normal walking, slow walking, fast walking, and normal walking with a bag), all in night conditions.

3.2. Radar Systems

Radar sensors could make it possible to monitor and analyze gait outside the laboratory and capture information about human gait during a person's everyday activities. Multiple studies concerning gait analysis have used this non-contact sensor, especially over the last few years. Different types of radars have been used at operating frequencies varying between 1 GHz and 77 GHz [50]. The general mechanism of a radar system works as follows: The system uses electromagnetic waves to detect objects and determine their range, velocity, and angle [51]. First, a transmitter antenna sends out a wave, and when it reaches an object, the wave is reflected towards the receiver antenna. Then, the receiver antenna picks up the returned signals. The use of a radar system is appealing due to its reliable functionality at different illumination levels, protection of privacy, penetration through obstacles, and long-range

---

[6] Skin colouration caused by the presence of melanin.
[7] Percentage of visible light that is reflected from the surface of the skin.
[8] Percentage of a medium such as UV to pass through the outer skin.
[9] A machine learning algorithm where data points are plotted onto N-dimensional hyperspace and the maximum distance between data points of different classes is searched for. N represents the number of data dimensions.

detection capabilities. Table 3.1 lists different radar systems used for gait analysis, outlining their frequency ranges, monitored gait parameters, and accuracy in detecting movement patterns.

3.2.1. Continuous Wave (CW)

Some of the developed radars can output one or several spatiotemporal parameters, as shown by Yang et al. [52]. Two CW radars were used to measure the gait, in-phase and quadrature (I/Q) demodulation, and short-time Fourier transform (STFT)[10] followed by feature extraction, which allowed researchers to obtain feature vectors. The feature vectors are characteristic of humans and can further be tested with respect to other moving objects [51]. A simple, binary classifier was developed to identify the presence of a person based on the STFT of signals from a CW radar by Otero [53]. The STFT performed on received signals from motion provides information on the signal in both the time and frequency domains (spectrogram) [54]. A Fourier transform was performed on each bin of the STFT results to extract the cadence frequency. While the results were promising, all the results (from the spectrogram) were only visualized; more sophisticated techniques are needed to resolve the contributions to gait motion from body parts such as the arms, upper leg, lower leg, and foot. Another study used the CW radar to measure several gait parameters such as torso velocity, cadence, stride period, acceleration and deceleration of the leg during the initial and terminal swing, supporting time, symmetry between motion of the legs, and time of three swing phases [55]. Twenty participants were asked to walk in front of a single-antenna CW radar system with an operating frequency of 10.52 GHz. By analyzing the envelope of the spectrogram, the researchers were able to extract the gait parameters and find differences between male and female participants as well as healthy versus individuals with Parkinson's disease. Unfortunately, the paper was unable to establish the accuracy of the results as there was no comparison to a ground-truth radar system.

Another research paper that used the CW radar used an X-band frequency that was comparatively lower than that of the other papers [56]. Due to size, money, and other constraints, the experiment was conducted on an open field with a 30–50-meter distance between the participant and the radar. The radar

---

[10] Mathematical operation used to measure the sinusoidal frequency and phase content of a signal that changes over time periods.

could precisely capture the Doppler signals and therefore extract gait parameters such as moving, swinging, stepping, walking, and running. This research study detected characteristics of body parts such as the calves, trunk, arms, and legs. Despite using a low-cost and low-frequency radar, the researchers were able to obtain a high-resolution measurement using the micro-Doppler signals. A study by Ma et al. also used a CW radar operating at 4.2 GHz to accurately classify the motions of the target human without detecting interference from non-target motions [57]. The researchers tested four motions that included walking with one arm swinging, without swinging arms, both arms swinging, and running. The researchers were able to establish an overall average classification accuracy of 97.3%. When broken down into each parameter, the accuracy ranged between 95% and 100%, with the lowest accuracy being walking with both arms swinging and the highest being running.

A method of estimating biomechanical gait parameters was proposed by Saho et al. using monostatic CW Doppler radar data corresponding to trunk movement [58]. This leads to stable estimations when compared to the conventional method based on leg movements due to the received powers of trunk echoes being larger and more stable than those of legs. The accuracy of gait parameters was evaluated against motion capture data, and it was experimentally demonstrated that the accuracy was similar. The step time in both methods had an error of around 10 ms, the step length of the CW radar had an error of 10 millimeters, whereas the motion capture had an error of 100 millimeters. However, the swing time, along with the stance time, had an error of 10 ms in motion capture but 100 ms in the CW radar. A new approach using deep CNNs by fusing the camera and radar sensors was proposed by Shi et al. [59] for complex covariate conditions. An RGB camera and an mm-wave radar were used to collect data from 121 subjects, eight views, and three walking conditions. The study demonstrated that this setup can capture highly complementary information for gait recognition, alleviating errors, especially in complex covariate conditions caused by a single type of sensor.

3.2.2. Frequency Modulated Continuous Wave (FMCW)

Like the single-frequency CW radar, frequency-modulated continuous wave (FMCW) radars have unique advantages that differentiate them from other radar systems. These features include simultaneous detection of range and angle, which makes this type of radar suitable for a variety of applications

[60]. The major advantages of these radars are being low-cost and low-power. An autonomous gait speed estimation (A-GSE) system that utilizes FMCW to measure gait speed was used by Boroomand et al. [61]. The FMCW used in this study had an operating frequency of 24 GHz and was paired with a location tracker to eliminate signals from static objects. Fourteen participants were asked to walk on the GAITRite® system for five meters at varying speeds. The results of the study concluded that a maximum accuracy of 74% to 86% is present at low, normal, and high speeds with respect to the ground truth result of the GAITRite® mat. This study concluded that the A-GSE system is good at identifying fast gait speeds using a frequency of 24 GHz.

Four experiments were conducted by van Dorp and Groen [62] using a 9.68 GHz FMCW radar to measure cycle frequency and cycle length. The researchers used two walker groups in which participants moved their arms and two stroller groups in which the participants' arms hung by their sides. They found different walking behaviours between the two groups and found that walkers had a greater cycle frequency than strollers. Furthermore, they found differences between the cycle lengths of the two walkers and equivalent cycle lengths for the two strollers. The average relative error for all four experiments was 7% for the variance in the fit function, 3% for the variance in the cycle length and frequency, and 2% for the variance in the cycle frequency based on the slope of the phase. A 77 GHz FMCW radar was used in a study where outdoor experiments were conducted to extract 3D spatial coordinates and radial velocity to classify jogging, squatting/standing, normal walking, and what they labelled lame walking, which is a combination of normal walking with one leg and the other dragging behind and arms slightly swinging [50]. The radar was able to accurately recognize the movements 88–93% of the time, with the least accurate being lame walking and the most accurate being normal walking. Another research study developed the WiGait sensor, which uses the FMCW radar to extract walking speed and stride length through the change in the position of the target [63]. The accuracy of the measures extracted from WiGait was assessed by comparing them to the Vicon system. Among the 18 subjects who participated in these experiments, the average error rates were 1.9% and 4.2% for gait velocity and stride length, respectively. Although this study obtained the overall velocity from the change in position, which is independent of the direction, all obtained parameters were average values. For instance, the stride length was extracted by the division of gait velocity by the stride frequency; this is an approximation rather than a true measured value. It is important to know the gait parameters for each cycle because the variation and instability of gait parameters during walking cycles can be obtained through the comparison between parameters extracted at each cycle. Moreover, their heuristic method to identify gait cycles and discriminate them from other activities will fail in the case of other periodic motions, for instance, a walking dog in the room.

A cloud-based in-home activity recognition and walking period identification system was introduced by Abedi et al. [64], using mm-wave FMCW radar sensors and sequential deep learning. The system could accurately identify walking periods and report on activity levels and other parameters. The deep GRU[11] network achieved 93% accuracy for known subjects and 87% for new subjects performing in-home activities. This system used a complex radar system including four AWR1243[12] chips to create 192 channels to provide human point cloud information for 2D-DCNN. A simpler and faster algorithm for real-time everyday use was designed by Abedi et al. [65]. For this solution, only one AWR1443Boost[13] radar sensor was used. Using the mm-wave radar system, human spectrograms (time-varying micro-Doppler patterns) were used to train deep Gated Recurrent Network (GRU) to identify physical activities performed by subjects in their living environment. An overall model accuracy of 93% was achieved to classify in-home physical activities.

A simple and cost-effective method was displayed in a 2022 paper, which extracted the subjects' gait parameters in a long hallway using a single FMCW radar [66]. It was demonstrated that unsupervised machine learning with a proposed tracking algorithm was able to track a subject in a long hallway and extract spatiotemporal gait parameters. A new method of noncontact gait analysis using MIMO FMCW was shown by Wang et al. [67]. A notable point of the study was that the MIMO radar types were shown to be able to differentiate between right and left legs and detect gait asymmetry with high accuracy. The accuracy was evaluated using 15 participants, wherein the received signals were preprocessed to obtain data on velocity, range, and angle. The correlation of gait parameters was high between the MIMO FMCW and IMU sensors. A gait classification solution for human identification and human-type recognition using a 60 GHz FMCW radar was proposed by Niazi et al. [68]. It used the cadence velocity being fed into the Gaussian prototypical network for classification and demonstrated better accuracy (3–4% increase) compared to the conventional CNN models with a dataset of 2080 recordings.

---

[11] A Gated Recurrent Unit is a gating mechanism in recurrent neural networks, used to better remember patterns in a series of data.
[12] 76-GHz to 81-GHz high-performance automotive monolithic microwave integrated circuit.
[13] 76-GHz to 81-GHz automotive radar sensor that uses a single chip.

Another approach for extracting the spatiotemporal gait values of people walking in hallways was shown by Abedi et al. [69]. An in-package hyperbola-based dielectric lens antenna was designed and integrated with a radar module package. This particular work was designed for single-subject tracking. This dielectric lens was paired with a MIMO FMCW radar [70]. The proposed system achieved around 14 dB gain improvements compared to the stand-alone radar module. It was validated by capturing spatiotemporal gait values in a highly reflective hallway.

3.2.3. Impulse-Radio Ultra-Wide Band (IR-UWB)

An Ultra-Wide Band (UWB)-based full-body capture system has been proposed by di Renzo et al. [71]. It uses Impulse Radio Ultra-Wide Band (IR-UWB) technology that captures impulses to generate gait measures. In a study using this technology, two IR-UWB radar sensors were installed on a 1.5-meter stand in a large area [72]. The radar was able to count the people who were simultaneously walking through a passage. In this paper, the IR-UWB was primarily used to count the number of people as opposed to capturing their location. Other research studies used the IR-UWB to extract motion and shape measures. In one of these studies, participants used a treadmill at a speed of 3 km/h, and the antennas were placed 2.7 meters from the participants' torso [73]. Through this experiment, the researchers were able to collect measures such as walking cycle, walking steps, shoulder width, and height. They were also able to collect data on walking motion, such as swinging of arms and radial velocity. Similarly, one study used an IR-UWB radar with a frequency range of 3.1 GHz to 5.3 GHz to extract gait parameters such as walking speed, leg orientation, and distance travelled [74]. The researchers were also among the first to extract gait measures from physiological processes such as breathing and heart rate, along with arm swing. They found that it can be done; however, the radar threshold to detect physiological movement needs to be done through an experimental approach since a higher or lower value may detect unwanted movement. They conducted the experiments in two settings, one in an anechoic chamber and the other in a real environment, and compared their data to a Samsung Health smartphone application to validate the findings. The validation results indicated that in both environments, compared to the smartphone application, the results varied within 5% of each other, indicating high validity of the results. The IR-UWB radar, compared to a ground truth system such as the GAITRite® mat, is also promising. In a 2018 study, six participants were asked to walk at varying speeds over a 5-meter distance. When comparing the accuracy of the UWB radar to GAITRite®, they found that the radar had an accuracy rate between 85% and 96% [75].

3.2.4. Pulse-Doppler Ultra-Wide Band (UWB)

Within the same scope, a study from Wang and Fathy had a pulse-Doppler radar using UWB technology to assess the time, frequency, and range of multiple people and through walls [76]. The study's participants were asked to walk behind a cement wall (1 centimeter thick) at varying speeds and directions. During the experiment, the radar was placed 1 meter away from the wall and produced a high-range resolution that helped to differentiate between targets using the wideband pulse signal inside. The study also tested the radars' ability to detect Doppler frequency, which is effective at providing accurate measures for both high-resolution range profiles and Doppler information.

Another paper studied the pulse-Doppler radar's applications to a home environment to assess step time and walking speed [77]. The radar used had a frequency of 5.8 GHz and a range of 20 to 50 feet. The results from this radar were compared to the ground truth system for gait analysis, Vicon. The 13 participants in this study were asked to walk at varying speeds over 17 feet. The researchers placed the radar in two ways: the first on the ground to assess foot motion accurately, and the second on the ground and another at a 1.25-meter height to accurately capture torso movement. The results suggested that the pulse-Doppler radar captured a walking speed that was less than the Vicon. The relationship was expressed as Radar = 0.87 * Vicon. However, the ICC scores of 0.97 for the foot walking speed and 0.99 for the torso walking speed have good consistency. Regarding step recognition, similar results were observed, as the ICC score of 0.97 also indicated a high level of consistency. The pulse-Doppler radar was compared to the Vicon system to determine the validity of the radar's gait feature extraction [78]. The study found that the radar can accurately track gait velocity, mean stride duration, and variability compared to the ground truth system. The research concluded that similar trends were visible between both systems, and there was high accuracy and a considerably high error rate. Unfortunately, they were unable to provide concrete accuracy and error rates.

Table 3.1. Types of radar systems

Reference	Type of Radar System	Frequency of the Radar System	Monitored Gait Parameters	Accuracy of Results
[56, 52, 51, 53, 54, 55, 57, 59]	Continuous Wave (CW)	24 GHz	Step rate Mean velocity Torso velocity Stride period Cadence Acceleration of leg in initial swing and deceleration of leg in terminal swing Supporting time Time of 3 swing phase Measure of the symmetry between motion of legs.	Average classification accuracy rate is 97.3% Recognition accuracy rate of running is up to 100% Accuracy of walking without any arm swinging is 98% Accuracy of walking with one arm swinging is 96%. Accuracy of walking with both arms swinging is 95%
[50, 61, 62, 63, 82, 66, 67, 68, 64, 69, 83, 65, 84, 70, 85, 86]	Frequency Modulated Continuous Wave (FMCW)	5.6 GHz–81 GHz	Cycle frequency Cycle length Gait velocity Stride length Step count	Maximum accuracy of 74% to 86% is present from low, normal, and high speeds Jogging, normal walking and squatting/standing had an average accuracy rate of more than 92%. Accuracy of gait velocity is between 96.0% and 99.8% for gait velocity Accuracy of stride length is between 88.4% and 99.3% Accuracy of identifying walking periods is 100% with a precision accuracy of 95.7% Accuracy of identifying walking periods is 100% with a precision accuracy of 95.7% Accuracy of IoT-based recognition system is 93% for scenarios of known subjects

Reference	Type of Radar System	Frequency of the Radar System	Monitored Gait Parameters	Accuracy of Results
[71, 72, 73, 74, 75]	Impulse-Radio Ultra-Wide Band (IR-UBW)	3.1 GHz–10 GHz	Cadence Stride length Walking cycle Walking step Walking speed Lower limb orientation Step frequency Distance walked Shoulder width and height Swinging of arms Radial velocity	Overall variation of results compared to smartphone applications are within 5%. Accuracy of a fast speed is 85% to 93% Accuracy of a normal speed is 90% to 94% Accuracy of a slow speed is 90% to 96%
[76, 77, 78, 79, 80, 81]	Pulse-Doppler Ultra-Wide Band (UWB)	5.8 GHz–16.5 GHz	Gait velocity Stride duration Frequency of Walks Walking speed Detect falls	Accuracy of detecting walks is 91.8% The correlation between the gait speeds produced by the radar and Vicon system is 0.9788.

A 5.8 GHz pulse-Doppler radar was used to determine the frequency of walks in a normal living setting by Phillips et al. [79]. Experiments consisted of walking measures such as varying walking speeds and non-walking measures such as standing, dropping items, etc. The radar was able to detect walks most of the time with an accuracy of 91.8%, indicating promising results for an in-home gait monitoring system. Another study compared the pulse-Doppler radar to the Vicon system to validate its ability to detect gait speed [80]. Ten participants were asked to walk across a 15-foot-long strip at a slow, usual, and fast pace. The results from this study were promising as well and produced a correlation of 0.98 when comparing the gait speed of the radar to the Vicon system. A radar sensor system that uses a segmentation approach to gait analysis has also been proposed [81]. The system automatically partitioned the walking pattern into phases (i.e., turning and walking straight) and evaluated the instantaneous gait speed of each phase. It then automatically segmented each walking phase into acceleration, normal, and deceleration parts. This segmentation process was validated using a Vicon system with 22 participants and a combined total of 396 signals. Its primary advantage was that these zones and phases were automatically determined without needing additional time, space, or synchronization.

3.3. Contact Devices for Gait Analysis

Several contact device forms, such as wearables and Inertial Measurement Units (IMU) sensors, have been designed to collect data for gait analysis. These devices are directly connected to the person of interest, either straight to the body or as an attachment to the person. This section aims to disclose several available contact devices used to monitor gait.

3.3.1. Wearables and Inertial Measurements Units (IMU) Sensors

Multiple IMUs exist and have been used for gait analysis. However, as has been demonstrated in several publications, not all of them are as reliable as GAITRite® or validated systems. Although IMU sensors are non-invasive, they require patients to wear them to obtain data. Additionally, the lack of standardized protocols and results can present problems when gathering or comparing data from the IMU [87]. The location or presence of the sensor disturbing the patients and changing their gait is another issue.

Technologies Available for Gait Analysis

IMUs can be composed of one-, two-, or three-axis accelerometers, magnetometers, gyroscopes, GPS sensors, or barometers. Wearable sensors have been developed for gait analysis because of their ease of use and the fact that full-body motion can be obtained for those that are wireless. Moreover, data can be obtained from inside or outside environments. IMU sensors can also be used for fall detection [88].

There are multiple examples of IMU wearable sensors for gait analysis, one of which is the BTS G-WALK®, composed of a triaxial accelerometer, a triaxial gyroscope, and a triaxial magnetometer [89]. The BTS G-Walk® is a sensor that must be worn in a belt on the fifth lumbar spine vertebrae, and the user can walk a 60-meter distance in the light-of-sight Bluetooth® range of the device [89]. The validity of this wearable sensor has been investigated by Ridder et al. by comparing it to the GAITRite® system [90]. Researchers have measured 30 healthy participants' spatiotemporal gait parameters (speed, cadence, stride length and duration, stance and swing time, double and single support) with both the BTS G-WALK® and the GAITRite® systems. They concluded that this sensor was reliable for the spatiotemporal gait parameters of healthy participants, and its validity was excellent for speed, stride length, duration, and cadence. However, the validity of the parameters based on final foot contact displayed lower levels of accuracy. The BTS G-WALK® has also been used in research to analyze the gait of older adults [91]. The effects of ranging physical activity for older adults were monitored; thirty-four participants wore a G-Sensor® so that the gait speed, stride and gait cycle duration, stance, swing, and double phase duration were acquired. The study concluded that gait parameters and sit-to-stand (STS) improved significantly during the vigorous physical activity group (VPA) compared to the light physical activity group (LPA). LPA showed some signs of a reduction in the swing phase, but the physical activity contributed to the general reduction of postural sway overall.

Another existing IMU-based sensor is the Physilog sensor by MindMaze Group SA [92]. The sensor consists of a 3D accelerometer, a 3D gyroscope, a 3D magnetometer, and a barometric pressure sensor, as per Table 3.2. The ranges and sample frequencies of this device are programmable. The sensors can be attached to each shoe or clipped to a belt or any other location, and the corresponding software, Census, can be used to process the data and analyze functional tests to estimate spatiotemporal gait parameters. This software allows users to obtain over 40 gait spatiotemporal parameters such as speed, cadence, stride length and time, and symmetry. For each parameter, a colour code, allowing the user to interpret their data values, is utilized. The Physilog system was first developed as a wireless 6D inertial measurement platform and has been respectfully developed and evaluated as a system [93]. The validation was realized against a pressure-insole system on 17 older adults. The specificity of the algorithm was 100%, and the sensitivity was 93.2% in detecting gait phases. The sensor performance was assessed by measuring the loss of signal frames, and experimental results showed that the overall performance was good for forwarding gait (1.2% loss) and side walking (0.3% loss). The validity of Physilog has also been investigated in several publications, one being by Mariani et al. [94]. A wireless sensor was attached to each foot of each of the 20 participants. The data's validity and accuracy were determined by comparing the IMU values to the optical motion capture[14]. The measured parameters determined at each gait cycle were stride length, stride velocity, foot clearance, and turning angle. The repeatability of the measurements for the system was also assessed. The results after the analysis of 974 cycles showed the mean accuracy was 1.5 ± 6.8 centimeters for stride length, 1.4 ± 5.6 cm/s for stride velocity, 1.9 ± 2.0 centimeters for foot clearance, and 1.6 ± 6.1° for turning angle. The accuracy of these results is further supported by the ranges of 0.04–0.06 m/s for gait speed. Despite the small magnitude of these results within this range, gait speed measurements are most likely detectable and ideal for clinical practice [95].

It was determined that inertial sensors' signals (Physilog) provided greater accuracy when compared to a reference standard by Mariani et al. [96], who assessed the foot-flat and stance phases of patients with ankle osteoarthritis. Forty-two subjects wearing a single sensor on a foot and pressure insoles as a reference had to perform a 50-meter walk. A dataset of 3193 gait cycles was then used to compare the IMU values to the pressure insole values. Heel-strike, toe-strike, heel-off, and toe-off were measured to estimate values of absolute and relative stance periods: loading response, foot-flat, and push-off. The limit of agreement values were computed using standard deviation, resulting in the percentage of stance periods: -0.6%–1.8% for Load, 1.3%–4.7% for Foot-flat, and -3.6%–0% for Push. Overall, these percentages showed a good consensus for IMU values (Physilog) and the reference values. This research demonstrated that the Physilog sensors are accurate and precise, with the average (mean ± standard deviation) error being -16 ± 13 ms for push phases and 19 ± 14 ms for foot-flat phases. Moreover, Physilog has also been validated in physical medicine for patients with Duchenne muscular

---

[14] The use of multiple cameras to determine the 3-dimensional position of a certain marker.

dystrophy[15], patients with Parkinson's disease, patients recovering from major surgeries for ankle osteoarthrosis, and patients with cerebral palsy graded GMFCS[16] I and II [97]- [98]. MINDMAZE, GAITUP, and PHYSILOG are trademarks of MindMaze Group SA registered in various countries.

The APDM Wearable Technologies brand has created Opal sensors that can be used with the Mobility Lab™[17] software to conduct gait analysis [99], [100]. The Opal sensor comprises a 6G accelerometer to measure low acceleration, a 200-m/s^2 accelerometer to measure dynamic movement, a 2000-°/s gyroscope, a magnetometer, and a barometer. Several Opals can be used on only one network, and the raw kinematic data is accessible and can be streamed to MATLAB, Java, Python, and C. Various studies have been conducted using the Opal sensor to collect data from participants wearing the sensor. The validity of the Mobility Lab™ has been assessed by comparing the obtained values from GAITRite® data [101]. Fifty-seven participants wore three sensors, one strapped to the lumbar spine and one on both feet, and they had to walk on the GAITRite® mat. The measured parameters were gait velocity, stride length, cadence, stride time, swing time, single support, double support, stride length variability, and stride time variability. The ICC was used to assess the validity of the Mobility Lab™ [102]. The ICC was higher than 0.75 for the gait velocity, the stride length, the cadence, the stride length, time variability, and the stride time, but was lower for swing time (ICC = 0.517), single support (ICC = 0.528), and double support (ICC = 0.518). Thus, the system is not as reliable as GAITRite®, especially for temporal parameters. The validity of the Opal sensors has also been assessed in collecting gait parameters [101]. Thirty-nine participants wore sensors on both feet and ankles while walking on an instrumented treadmill[18] for validation or on the ground and the split-belt treadmill[19] for testing repeatability. This study demonstrated that the sensor was accurate and repeatable for spatiotemporal gait parameters. The Opal sensors have also been used to research Parkinson's disease [103]. The research aimed to develop models of gait and balance for patients with Parkinson's disease and to determine the gait and balance characteristics related to cognition. Six Opal IMUs were used for a 2-minute

---

[15] A genetic disorder that progressively causes muscle degeneration and weakness.
[16] Gross Motor Function Classification System: categories children based on their abilities and limitations regarding cerebral palsy.
[17] A portable laboratory, to collect and store assessments for gait; data analysis can be done based on the collected data.
[18] A type of treadmill that allows for data to be recorded or captured from the participant's usage.
[19] A type of treadmill where the belt is split, allowing for each belt to run at different speeds or directions.

continuous walk on the 198 participants to assess gait. The six sensors were placed on the wrist, the feet, the sternum, and the L5[20]. The Mobility Lab™ was used for the analysis of the gait parameters. These sensors have also been used for gait analysis in a 2019 study to investigate movement coordination while walking in a complex topological arrangement using nine participants [104]. The sensor was placed at the back of the participants' necks, at the level of the 7th cervical vertebra, and only the vertical component of the acceleration was used. Ten participants wore two Opal sensors on their trunk and right shank in another study designed to evaluate the minimal number of strides and within-session reliability [105]. This was done to obtain stride time and variability measures related to stride time to determine the minimum number of required strides for gait analysis. The Opal IMU has also been utilized to obtain the stride length, stride time, stride velocity, cadence, stance phase percentage, peal sagittal and frontal plane trunk velocity for research investigating the impact of a treadmill on gait analysis [106]. A p-value greater than 0.05 was used for all comparisons in this study to determine the significance of the measurements. The study concluded that after the comparison of the mean values of the spatiotemporal gait parameters, there was no significant (a p-value of less than 0.05) difference between the overground and treadmill conditions. Short-term variability and long-term variability indicators for gait analyzed on the treadmill were significantly (p-value higher than 0.05) reduced in relation to the values gathered from overground walking. The article further stated that the treadmill ambulation has a less varied gait, thereby implying that invariant gait patterns on treadmills could impact a person's capacity to use their locomotor skills gained through training on the treadmill and apply them to overground situations [106].

The Free4Act is an IMU sensor developed in 2007 by LetSense Group [107]. It is composed of a triaxial accelerometer, a triaxial gyroscope, and a triaxial magnetometer. A data logger unit allows the user to control between one and sixteen sensors together. The data from these sensors can be interpreted with the Biomech® software[21]. The sensors have been used to obtain step and stride duration, step and stride length, speed, cadence, symmetry, stance and swing time, and single and double duration [108]. For this research, only the 3-axial accelerometer was used, and another software

---

[20] The 5th vertebrae of the lumbar spine.
[21] Analysis software for kinetics and 3D kinematics using visuals.

Technologies Available for Gait Analysis 33

(BioActiStudio[22]) was used to analyze the data. The sensor was placed over the L4-L5 intervertebral space with a semi-elastic belt. With a level of significance lower than 0.05, the results of the study indicated that despite improvements in certain individuals, the entirety of the group did not show significant improvement (lower than 0.05 for the majority of categories). It was only determined for MS patients in two categories: Step pathological foot [m] – p-value: 0.01 and Step healthy foot [m] – p-value: 0.03; both values were under the 0.05 threshold, and hence were significant improvements. In conclusion, despite the limited improvements to patients, AFO[23] may still be useful in preliminary results of rehabilitation outcomes.

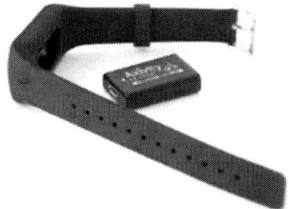

Figure 3.7. AX3 sensor [109].

Another example is the AX3 sensor from Axivity, which is a 3-axial accelerometer (Figure 3.7, courtesy of Axivity Limited) [109]. Its accuracy has been investigated by comparing it to the GAITRite® system by Godrey et al. [110]. The participants wore a sensor on their L5, and the measurements were realized while participants were walking on the GAITRite® walkway. The parameters analyzed were step time, stride time, stance time, swing time, step length, and step velocity. The ICC and the p-value were calculated, and it was demonstrated that the ICC was sufficient for the mean spatiotemporal values (level of agreement was 0.969 for YHP; 1.00 for OHP, where $p < 0.05$) but poor for the variability and the symmetry [110]. The validity of the system has also been assessed by Del Din et al. [111]. Fourteen gait characteristics: the mean, variability, and asymmetry of step time, stance time, swing time, and step length, and the mean and variability of the velocity were measured for 30 participants with an Axivity sensor and a GAITRite® walkway. The ICC was excellent for four parameters (0.913–0.983), moderate for four other parameters (0.508–0.766), and poor for six parameters (0.637–0.370). From

---

[22] Software that allows for data analysis and visualisation, through filters, sampling frequency, and adjusting accelerometer sensibility.

[23] Ankle-foot orthosis (AFO) is a wireless inertial device to measure gait parameters.

the study, it was concluded that the Axivity sensors are not accurate enough for gait analysis because the gait sensor/monitor captures more sensitive data for asymmetry and variability features; hence why ICC values were poorer for these characteristics. The Axivity sensors were also investigated for the influence of device location and testing protocol for measuring gait with an accelerometer [112]. Eighty participants, who were grouped by age into older adults (OA) and younger adults (YA), wore the sensors at the chest, waist, and lower back. Then, the mean, variability, and asymmetry gait characteristics were calculated from the sensor data. The chest was an excellent location for mean step time and length, moderate for step time and length asymmetry in relation to L5 (lower back) ($ICC_{2,1} > 0.886$). The waist was an excellent location for mean step time and good for mean step length (YA: $ICC_{2,1} > 0.928$ for step time/length) (OA: $ICC_{2,1} > 0.981$ for step time, $ICC_{2,1} = 0.589$ for step length) in relation to L5 (lower back) [112]. For variability, chest step time had a moderate ICC for OA ($ICC_{2,1} = 0.513$), while YA had poor ICC ($ICC_{2,1} < 0.394$); the waist for both OA/YA had poor ICC ($ICC_{2,1} < 0.285$). Lastly, for asymmetry, the chest for both OA/YA had good ICCs ($ICC_{2,1} > 0.582$), whereas the waist ICC for both OA/YA was poor ($ICC_{2,1} < 0.529$). Overall, the mean spatiotemporal gait parameters measured were highly accurate in comparison to the variability and asymmetry.

The DynaPort MoveMonitor sensor is a 3-axial gyroscope that can be used with the DynaPort software to obtain information about gait [113]. The validity of the DynaPort software was assessed using DynaPort sensors [114]. The reference method was a video recording of patients walking. Fourteen participants walked several times in a straight corridor, and parameters including the number of steps, step time (for the intact and prosthetic leg), step length, and walking speed were analyzed. The statistics calculated for each parameter included the absolute mean difference, the relative mean difference, the PCC, and the p-value. The PCC was higher than 0.98 for the walking speed, the step length, and the number of steps, with a p-value of less than 0.001. Hence, the system is valid for assessing the spatiotemporal parameters of gait, but not reliable since the PCC is 0.82 (with a p-value of 0.01) for the step time of prosthetic and intact heel strikes. Moreover, the DynaPort sensor has been used in research, and with an accuracy of parameters within 6.5%, the DynaPort shows good reliability and validity for its use in gait analysis. A DynaPort IMU sensor was also used to determine the walking speed, the stride time, and the coefficient of variation of the stride time [115].

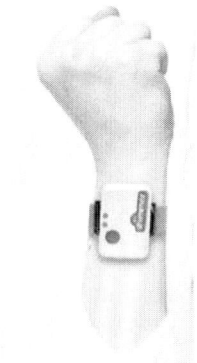

Figure 3.8. Shimmer 3 [116].

Shimmer3, as shown in Figure 3.8, is also an IMU sensor that has been used for gait analysis [116]. Research from 2018 has compared the reliability of a single Shimmer3 with a ground truth composed of a pair of FootMoov[24] 2.0 shoes and two Shimmer3 devices [117]. The FootMoov 2.0 shoes are composed of five sensors, and the Shimmer3 devices are composed of an ST-Micro tri-axial accelerometer, a digital magnetometer, a gyroscope, and a pressure/temperature sensor. The test of reliability for a single wearable sensor was realized for two positions: over the lower trunk and inside a trouser pocket. Three volunteers were asked to perform two 40-meter walks on level ground, and the results were that trunk and pocket positions had a mean absolute error below 50 ms for estimating the studied gait parameters (stride time, swing, and stance duration). Shimmer sensors were also used alone for gait analysis [118]. The research aimed to compare the performance of the algorithms for the Shimmer sensor with the performance of GAITRite® for heel-strike, toe-off, stride time, swing time, stance time, stride length, and velocity. The ICC was used to assess the validity of the data of the seven participants. The ICCs were more than 0.84 for the temporal parameters and more than 0.88 for the spatial gait parameters. Hence, with the used algorithms, the accuracy of the sensor is comparable to the GAITRite® accuracy.

---

[24] A type of wearable shoe device that allows for the capture of biometric data through sensors.

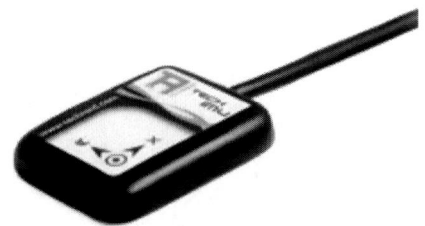

Figure 3.9. CV4 sensor [119].

Two sensors from Technaid, the Tech IMU CV4 and the Tech IMU V4, are IMUs that can be used for gait analysis with the Mobility Lab™ software (Figure 3.9, Figure 3.10) [119]. Both sensors are composed of a 3D accelerometer, a 3D gyroscope, and a 3D magnetometer. The two sensors are similar and could be used for gait analysis; the difference is that the IMU CV4 is more robust and waterproof. The sensors can be worn on any part of the body since it is a wireless system, weighing less than 15 grams. In 2015, a Technaid SL sensor was used in two studies: one for monitoring the differences seen in varying ages when walking on specific terrains [120], and one for gender-related characteristics for gait [121]. Fifty-seven participants in the first study and 122 in the second had sensors positioned in the pelvis area and at the posterior part of the head with elastic bands. The parameters calculated were walking speed, cadence, step length, step time variability, acceleration root mean square, attenuation, and harmonic ratio. The main findings of the former study indicated that older adults adjust to a more conservative gait (slow speed, shorter steps, increased cadence), which has been related to increased fall risk [122]. The main findings of the latter study indicated important gender differences in gait, spatiotemporal, and quality parameters. Although the men and women walked at the same speed, women walked with a faster cadence and shorter steps than men.

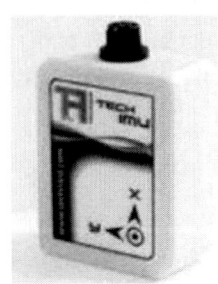

Figure 3.10. V4 sensor [119].

MicroStone Inc.[25] has developed an IMU using a combination of an accelerometer, a gyroscope, and a magnet attachment [123]. The system outputs the location and orientation of the device in 3D space. This data can be used to record rehabilitation, sports motion, and analyze some gait parameters. The sensor was used to obtain the lower leg proximal end and forefoot kinematics by Wang et al. [124]. The participants had to walk on a treadmill at paces of 5 km/h and 9 km/h, and their gait cycles were also recorded with a video camera. The data obtained was compared with statistical software (PASW[26] Statistics 18.0). The values derived from the results concluded that the lower leg proximal end and forefoot maximum inversion/eversion (LL I/E and F I/E) rotation and medial/lateral (LL M/L and F M/L) rotation paces from 5 km/h and 9 km/h were reliable due to the intra-examiner reliability. In intra-examiner reliability, these estimates indicate that for (LL I/E) and (LL M/L) rotation, it ranged from 0.82–0.89 and 0.87–0.93, whereas for (F I/E) and (F M/L), it ranged from 0.92–0.84 and 0.93–0.91. This research demonstrated that the MVP-RF8-BC[27] IMU was reliable for the measurement of lower leg proximal end and forefoot kinematics. The MVP-RF8-BC was also used in a 2014 study to measure walking speed, cadence, percentage of swing time, and stride length [125]. The outcome of the study was that, in comparison to the usual condition, the fast-paced condition's decreased toe flexor strength was significantly linked to slower walking speed (p = 0.049), shorter stride length (p = 0.011), and lower percent swing time in the gait cycle (p = 0.009); all these values were lower than 0.05 (the threshold for p-value), meaning that they were significant. Therefore, the results of this study indicate the importance of toe flexor muscles for gait in older individuals.

Another IMU-based method for gait analysis is using miniature piezoelectric gyroscopes[28], as performed by Aminian et al. [126]. Another study measured the gait of 20 participants with three miniature piezoelectric gyroscopes (Murata, ENC-03J), all attached to the patient's right thighs, and with foot pressure sensors[29] as a reference [127]. The analyzed parameters were velocity, stride length, duration of the gait cycle, left and right stance, and the initial and terminal double support. There were no significant

---

[25] A company that developed an Inertial Measurement Unit (IMU) to obtain 3D motion and gait analysis.
[26] Statistical software used to perform data analysis and management.
[27] Wireless Motion Recorder, an IMU device that was produced by MicroStone Inc.
[28] A device used to detect movement on an axis that is perpendicular to the axis of rotation.
[29] A sensor that can analyse the individual's foot pressure distribution between their foot and their shoe.

differences in the toe-off detection, the stride length, or the gait velocity, but a systematic delay of 10 ms on average was present for heel strikes obtained by a foot pressure sensor or gyroscope. The error for velocity was 0.06 m/s and the error for stride length was 0.07 m; thereby, minimal error estimations show the reliability and validity of the Murata. Hence, the Murata could have applications in rehabilitation, gait analysis, and fall risk estimation. Murata ENC-03J gyroscopes were also used for gait analysis in a 2005 paper [128]. The gyroscope was part of an IMU that also contained a bi-axial accelerometer (ADXL210E). The IMU was placed on the instep of the right foot and attached to the shoe. Five healthy adult males had to walk on a treadmill on which speed and incline could be adjusted. The studied parameters were walking speed, stride time, duration of the swing phase, duration of the stance phase, and relative stance. Footswitches[30] were used as a reference by placing them underneath the heel of the big toe. Their output was coordinated with the IMU signals, allowing both the time of heel-strike and toe-off to be measured. After 300 gait cycles, it was determined that IMU tends to detect signals 35 ms faster for toe-off, and the heel-strike is detected without any systematic difference, on average at -2 ms. It was concluded that this IMU was reliable and accurate for assessing walking speed and incline.

The IDEEA® (Intelligent Device for Energy Expenditure and Physical Activity) system developed by MiniSun[31] is another way to analyze gait [129]. The system consists of five bi-axial accelerometers placed on the feet, thighs, and sternum, connected with a data logger worn on the waistband. MiniSun has also developed the software ActView (GaitView)™, which allows users to access information about their posture, gait, and activity during measurements. The validity of this system was assessed by Rigsby [130], and the reference was the Opal IMU from APDM. The research analyzed the gait of 32 subjects. A p-value higher than 0.05 was used to determine if there was a significant difference between the value measured by the Opal sensor and the IDEEA sensor. It was shown that there was a significant difference in gait speed, cadence, and step length, meaning that the accuracy of the IDEEA is not high enough for a gait analysis measurement.

---

[30] A device that is controlled by the participant's feet to switch the device in an on or off state.
[31] The company that developed IDEEA, a gait analysis system.

Table 3.2. Contact devices for gait analysis

Devices	Size (mm³)	Weight (g)	Features
BTS G-WALK [89]	70 x 40 x 18	37	Tri-axial accelerometer, gyroscope, magnetometer
Physilog [92]	26.5 x 47.5 x 10	11	3D accelerometer, 3D gyroscope and baromatic pressure sensor
AX3 [109]	23 x 32.5 x 7.6	11	3-axis accelerometer
V4 [119]	36 x 26 x 11	10	3D accelerometer, 3D gyroscope and 3D magnetometer
CV4 [119]	36 x 26 x 8	14	3D accelerometer, 3D gyroscope and 3D magnetometer
Opal [99]	43.7 x 39.7 x 13.7	25	2*3 axis accelerometer, 3 axis magnetometer and 3 axis gyroscope
MVP-RF8 [123]	45 x 45 x 18	60	3D accelerometer and 3D gyroscope
Dynaport [113]	106.6 x 58 x 11.5	55	3 axial gyroscope

3.3.2. Gait Analyses through Footwear and Insoles

The analysis of gait parameters in laboratories is a time-consuming process that requires frequent supervision of gait parameters and the patients in the study. In recent years, there have been many technological advancements in the insoles of footwear and their ability to capture data. Through precisely calibrated sensors, these insoles are able to gather the pressure distribution of a patient's foot, thereby providing gait analysis for stationary and walking movements.

Several models of shoes with embedded sensors have been developed because of their ease of use. For example, the FootMoov shoes have an IMU sensor with a 3D accelerometer, 3D gyroscope, and 3D magnetometer embedded within them, with microprocessors and a wireless module [131]. The IMU is better known as an inertial measurement unit in the case of these shoes: a single-point IMU is used alongside the accelerometer that gathers data to provide an accurate orientation along the X, Y, and Z axes [132]. The communication is obtained via Bluetooth, so that data from the shoes can be wirelessly controlled by a smartphone. In an article testing the accuracy of wearable sensors for gait analysis, it was determined that using a single accelerometer via footwear, foot contact, and temporal gait parameters could be detected without the need for supervision. The data was collected via a smartphone. The results of the study were that in terms of positions on the body, the trunk, pocket, and shoe conditions obtained similar results for the parameters of stride time, stance duration, and swing duration. Therefore, after completion of the Bland-Altman analysis, the mean difference between the shoe and trunk or the shoe and pocket position both had a mean difference of either 0.00 seconds or -0.01 seconds for the above three parameters. Hence, using gait devices in footwear has proved to be an effective method to collect accurate gait analysis data [117].

Another shoe-integrated wireless sensor system was created, analyzed, and explained by Bamberg et al. [133]. The system, named "GaitShoe," is composed of three orthogonal accelerometers, three orthogonal gyroscopes, four force sensors, two bidirectional blend sensors, two dynamic pressure sensors, and electric field height sensors. It can be worn in any shoe and costs under 500 USD per foot. After data transformation, the stride length and the velocity are determined by a double- and single-integration of the kinematic acceleration along the X_{room}-axis, respectively. The GaitShoe has been worn by ten healthy walkers and five Parkinsonian patients, and the data was sufficient to separate the two gait patterns. The parameters used to differentiate the gait patterns were maximum and minimum pitch[32], stride length, stride time, and percent stance time. The healthy people's gait range was much larger than that of the Parkinsonians'. The mean values of the maximum and minimum pitch were 14.5° and 7.5° beyond for the healthy persons, respectively. The normal stride length was a mean 0.26-meter length longer than the Parkinsonian stride length. Though the stride time of the normal subjects was shorter by 0.15 seconds, the percentage of the stride spent in stance was nearly equivalent, with the normal subjects spending only 2.2% less time in stance.

Insoles[33] that can be put in shoes have also been developed, like the FeetMe® insole in which pressure sensors and IMU are embedded [134]. The system works with a battery that lasts 24 hours, and the data can be transmitted through Bluetooth communication. The spatiotemporal parameters of gait obtained with those insoles are stride length, walking speed, width motion, cadence, stride time, swing time, single and double support time, stride length difference, stride time difference, and support asymmetry. FeetMe® can be used for evaluation, rehabilitation, and stimulation of gait. The validity and

---

[32] The pitch was determined by integrating the z-gyroscope output over single strides, from heel-strike to toe-off.
[33] A removable type of shoe sole that can be used to obtain qualitative data.

accuracy of FeetMe insoles for gait speed in stroke patients were analyzed by Farid et al. [135]. It was evident from the ICC values that the spatiotemporal parameters and the duration of the gait cycle phases both showed good reliability. The study concluded that for velocity, stride length, and cadence measurements (spatiotemporal parameters), ICC values were greater than 0.95. Hence, the validity was confirmed with a high degree of confidence. For the gait cycle phases on the paretic side, the stance duration (ICC > 0.77) and swing phase (ICC > 0.90) both showed good validity. It was only the non-paretic side, whereas the swing duration (ICC > 0.57) had moderate validity. Overall, the study concluded that FeetMe monitors are a great device for spatiotemporal gait analysis, especially outside the laboratory.

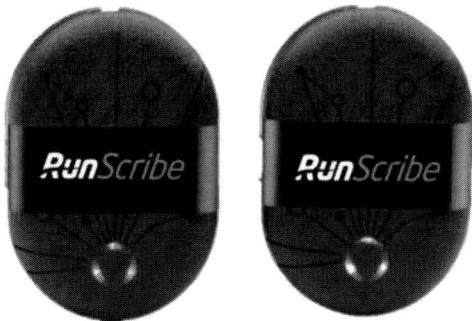

Figure 3.11. RunScribe devices [136].

Another example of insoles is the RunScribe® insoles with an embedded 9-axis motion sensor working with a phone app or computer dashboard to obtain gait parameters such as stride rate, contact time, or symmetry (Figure 3.11) [136]. The accuracy of RunScribe location on spatiotemporal gait characteristics was studied in a 2020 study [137]. It was shown that, in comparison to the high-speed video analysis system at 1000 Hz, the RunScribe was able to provide accurate measurements of spatiotemporal parameters. The ICC values showcased highly similar results between RunScribe and the high-speed video analysis: contact time/flight time (ICC 0.85–0.90), step length/step frequency (ICC 0.96–0.97), hence proving the reliability and validity of the RunScribe system's use in gait analysis.

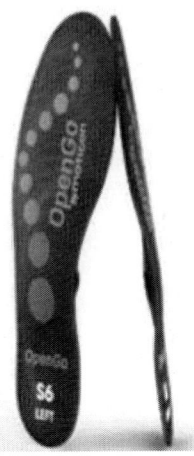

Figure 3.12. OpenGo insoles [138].

Furthermore, Moticon® has developed the OpenGo[34] insoles with 16 pressure sensors and a 6-axis gyroscope embedded, as shown in Figure 3.12 [138]. This system is made to be used with OpenGo Analyse software. OpenGo Analyse is one of the modules from the OpenGo software package that calculates the stance phase, the gait speed timing, the length and width of the gait line, the stance time, the cadence, and the double support time. The insoles have been demonstrated to be accurate [139]. The Zebris FDM-S System is a force-measuring plate that contains force sensors calibrated to measure and analyze the static and dynamic forces produced from stationary standing and walking movements [140]. This system was used as a reference for testing the reliability of the system on 12 participants and gait line length for right and left, gait line width for right and left, gait cycle time, cadence, double support time, stance left and right, and swing left and right. The ICC was used for the statistical analysis and was higher than 0.796 for temporal parameters, giving a fairly high degree of confidence in its validity.

3.3.3. Stride Analyzers

Stride analyzers are also systems that could be used for gait analysis. They are composed of a footswitch, two leg transmitters, and a microprocessor that interprets data from the footswitch into outcome walking parameters such as

---

[34] OpenGo is a type of insole used in shoes to measure gait parameters.

velocity, gait cycle, stride length, or single and double support. Different brands have developed different stride analyzers, such as B&L Engineering or Siemens Healthineers [141]. The validity of stride analyzers has been assessed by Beckwée et al. [142]. A stride analyzer 5.10 model from B&L Engineering Stride Analyzer was tested and compared to a 16-camera infrared optoelectronic video-based motion capture system. The parameters of interest were gait speed, cadence, stride length, gait cycle, single limb support right and left, swing phase right and left, stance phase right and left, and double limb support right and left. Bland-Altman plots, intra-class correlation coefficient (ICC), and standard error of measurement were used to examine the validity and test-retest of the stride analyzer. The test-retest analyses have good results, with ICC values between 0.805 and 0.949. The agreement between the stride analyzer and the Vicon system was also good for velocity, cadence, stride length, and gait cycle, with ICC values between 0.943 and 0.962.

Chapter 4

Pathological Implications of Gait

This chapter discusses the potential utility and applicability of employing gait monitoring devices as a predictive tool for various physiological pathologies. This topic is particularly germane for older individuals, who tend to be disproportionately susceptible to cardiovascular, neuro-cognitive, and motor degeneration, as well as other bodily morbidities [143]. Older adult age groups make up an increasingly large proportion of the industrialized world's population, amplifying the need to invest in boosting the financial and logistical capacity of clinical infrastructure in Canada and around the world [143]. Essential to these efforts is enhanced screening and diagnostic technology that can detect signs of emerging disease prior to clinical intervention, and this is where gait monitoring can play a potentially central role.

4.1. General Predictions from Gait

Most of the studies released after 2010 focused on one specific pathological group (e.g., cognitive function). On the other hand, most of the studies released before that year were more global and assessed the association between gait speed and adverse events or hospitalization. An example of that is a study from 2005, in which the walking speed of 102 healthy adults over 75 years old was measured using a stopwatch, and their health was studied over the two following years, as per Table 4.1 [144]. Experiments showed that people with a low speed (<0.7 m/s) had a higher relative risk of hospitalization, a requirement for a caregiver, and new falls with a relative risk of 5.4. The assessment of walking speed was thus sufficient to predict adverse events for healthy older people. However, the limitations of the study were that the sample size was too small and that the duration of the 24-month experiment was too short.

Other studies have demonstrated the association between slow gait speed and adverse events, such as the study in [145], which assessed the association between gait speed and readiness for home discharge (an important concern for clinicians). Several variables, including preoperative gait speed, anesthesia time, and heart rate, were measured for 664 individuals. Their gait speed was measured with a stopwatch used by the same examiner, and patients were instructed to walk a 20-foot (6.10-meter) distance. Gait speed was separated into two groups: lower or greater than 1.0 m/s. The odds ratio[35] of having an unplanned admission was 0.35 for participants whose speed was lower than 1.0 m/s, compared to those who had a speed greater than 1.0 m/s. Also, gait speed was independently associated with early home discharge readiness. Thus, a gait speed test can predict whether a patient is at risk for an unplanned admission, as per Table 4.1. An association between slow gait speed and poor health outcomes has also been established using a quarter-mile test. While most gait analyses are based on results derived from a short walk test, generally shorter than 10 meters, Newman et al. assessed the relationship between long-distance corridor walk performance and poor health outcomes such as mortality, cardiovascular disease, mobility limitation, and disability with a quarter-mile (around a 400-meter) walk [146]. The sample was comprised of 3075 community-dwelling adults aged between 70 and 79 from the Health, Aging, and Body Composition Study[36]. The participants were instructed to walk a quarter mile in ten laps, with a 2-minute break between each lap. Some individuals were unable to walk 400 meters, and the participants in this category had the highest risk of mortality, cardiovascular disease, mobility limitation, and mobility disability. For those who were able to walk 400 meters, the statistical analysis showed that an additional minute was associated with an adjusted hazard ratio[37] between 1.20 and 1.52 for mortality, cardiovascular diseases, mobility limitations, and disability. Thus, a reduction in walking speed is associated with a higher risk of mortality and prospective adverse health events.

Multiple studies have been conducted to highlight the decrease in mobility experienced by older adults. A group of Australian researchers performed a review of 48 studies that were centered on gait speed for a total of 7000 inpatients or outpatients[38] aged 70 or older [147]. For the usual pace, the gait speed was estimated at 0.58 m/s, and the maximum pace was 0.89 m/s. The mean gait speeds for patients who did and did not belong to acute care settings were compared. Participants who belonged to acute care settings had a gait

---

[35] Measure of relative probability. Odds ratio < 1 in this case, indicating lower odds of an unplanned admission with speed < 1.0 m/s.
[36] A study that aims to identify risk factors behind later-life loss of functionality.
[37] Ratio of event probabilities with risk exposure relative to baseline probabilities.
[38] Inpatient: care requiring hospitalization. Outpatient: care not requiring hospitalization.

speed of 0.46 m/s, whereas the ones that did not belong had a gait speed of 0.74 m/s, confirming that there is an association between health and gait speed. A review was conducted in 2012 to evaluate the reliability, responsiveness, and validity of different clinical walking and gait speed tests to help clinicians choose the most appropriate test [148]. Researchers focused on walking speed at the usual pace and the fastest pace of each participant. Eighty-six articles were reviewed and analyzed with a standard checklist. The study established that the usual walking pace was the most reliable for community-dwelling people and that walking speed at the usual and maximum pace was a valid method. However, according to their criteria, there was no study that could attest to the reliability of the maximum walking pace. Moreover, for both usual and maximum pace, few studies analyzed the responsiveness for walking speed, so they were not able to reach conclusions regarding responsiveness. The review concluded that the usual pace is a good indicator of health, but the evaluation of the maximum walking pace needs to be assessed further.

Also, in the research that analyzed self-reported walking parameters from a sample of 221 adults (with a mean age of 79.9 years), the statistical data analysis demonstrated that self-reported items related to gait, such as walking speed and difficulty, are better predictors of functional mobility performance relating to chair-rise, stance maintenance, and walking than other Epidemiologic Studies of the Elderly[39] (EPESE) self-report items[40] [149]. Self-reported walking ability may be the best predictor of overall functional mobility. However, self-reported data is not as precise as measured data, and the results may not be accurate. Furthermore, when the gait speed and the EPESE battery were considered for 487 adults aged 65 and older from a medical health maintenance organization (HMO) and Veterans Affairs (VA), the results did not align [150]. In fact, after the first 12 months of follow-up, a majority of the patients who had been hospitalized were slow walkers (<0.6 m/s). The EPESE test (studying the walking speed, the chair rise, and the tandem stand) and its performances were superior to gait speed when both the Probabilities of Repeated Admission (PRA) scale and the primary physician's hospitalization risk estimate were included. The major limitation of this study is the lack of data on hospitalization risk for a subset of subjects. A study realized in the Cardiovascular Health Study at the Pittsburgh site, established that stance time variability was an independent predictor of future mobility

---

[39] A series of longitudinal studies that was conducted to examine the health and well-being of older populations.
[40] Typically include information related to demographics, health status, behaviours, medication use, etc.

disability [19]. The definition given for mobility disease was having difficulties walking a half-mile (approximately 800 meters), and the 379 adults assessed had no disabilities at the baseline. Researchers used a 4-meter computerized walkway to measure the speed of the participants. Following an adjusted Cox proportional hazards model[41] for gait speed, it was demonstrated that an association existed only between stance time variability and walking disability; an increase in stance time variability was related to a higher incidence of mobility disabilities.

Data from 907 adults in the population-based KORA-Age study was analyzed by researchers in 2013, revealing that tests with fast speed or dual-task walking had the best performance to measure a decline in gait performance in age-related endoprosthesis and mobility aid analyses [21]. The decrease in gait parameters in these harder gait tasks may be attributed to a lack of resources for compensation among older adults. The participants were instructed to complete seven walking tasks: three at a different speed and four at normal speed with an additional task. The gait speed was measured with the electronic walkway system GAITRite®, and the large sample was enough to guarantee the validity of the statistical power for regression.

The principal purpose of the Baltimore Longitudinal Study of Aging was to determine whether there was an association between gait characteristics and walking speed [13]. Researchers have measured cadence, percent of the gait cycle in double stance, stride width, anterior-posterior mechanical work expenditure[42] (MWE), medial-lateral MWE, and stride length with a 3-dimensional motion capture system and force platform for the 362 participants with a mean follow-up time of 3.2 years. Gait speed was assessed at a 6-meter distance. The meaningful decline was defined as a reduction of 0.05 m/s/year in gait speed, and the parameters were evaluated with a logistic regression adjusted for age, sex, race, height, weight, initial walking speed, and follow-up time. Researchers concluded that faster cadence and longer strides were associated with lower odds of decline.

One study aimed to evaluate whether gait during challenging conditions could be a predictor of gait decline after one year [151]. The cohort was composed of 71 adults with a usual gait speed greater than 1.0 m/s at baseline, who had to walk under four different conditions: narrow walking, stepping over an obstacle, simple walking while talking, and complex walking while talking.

---

[41] A statistical regression model that is used to examine associations between predictor variables and the occurrence of events of interest.
[42] A kinetic and kinematic estimate of joint movement and power generation.

Table 4.1. Gait and general predictions

Study	Sample	Method of analysis	Duration of the follow-up	General predictions
Self-reported walking ability predicts functional mobility performance in frail older adults [77] (2000)	221 adults (mean age = 79.9 years)	Self-reported walking parameters	/	Walking speed is a better predictor than the EPESE battery
Physical performance measures in the clinical setting [78] (2003)	487 adults aged 65 and older	Stopwatch (four-meter walk)	1 year	Those who had been hospitalized were a majority of slow walkers (0.6 m/s)
Gait velocity as a single predictor of adverse events in healthy seniors aged 75 years and older [79] (2005)	102 participants aged over 75	Stopwatch (8 meter measured of a 10-meter walk)	2 years	Participants with a low speed (< 0.7 m/s) had higher relative risk of hospitalization (RR = 5.9), falls (RR = 5.4) and need for a caregiver (RR = 9.5)
Association of long-distance corridor walk performance with mortality, cardiovascular disease, mobility limitation, and disability [146] (2006)	3,075 community-dwelling individuals aged between 70 and 79	Stopwatch (400-meter walk in 10 laps)	Mean follow-up of 4.9 years	Individuals that were not able to walk 400 meters had the highest risk of all pathologies. A slower baseline speed was associated with high risk of pathologies
Challenging gait conditions predict 1-year decline in gait speed in older adults with apparently normal gait [80] (2011)	71 participants with a usual gait >1.0 m/S	Stopwatch (walks with challenging conditions (e.g., walking while talking or stepping over obstacles))	1 year	The participants whose speed declined had the highest walking speed at baseline and the best result at narrow walk and stepping over obstacle

Table 4.1. (Continued)

Study	Sample	Method of analysis	Duration of the follow-up	General predictions
Decline in fast gait speed as a predictor of disability in older adults [81] (2015)	3,814 individuals aged between 65 and 85	Two photoelectric cells connected to a chronometer	11 years	Accelerated decline in fast gait speed is associated with disabilities
Can a simple gait speed test predict ambulatory surgical discharge outcomes? [145] (2013)	664 participants after a surgery	Stopwatch (6.10-meter walk)	24 hours	Gait speed can predict the risk of unplanned rehospitalization after a surgery
Gait characteristics associated with walking speed decline in older adults: results from the Baltimore longitudinal study of aging [13] (2015)	362 participants aged 60 to 89	3-dimensional motion capture system and force platform	3.2 years	Faster cadence and longer strides are associated with lower odds of decline
Gait speed as a measure in geriatric assessment in clinical settings: a systematic review [147] (2013)	7,000 participants over 48 studies (literary review)	/	/	The mean walking speed of the participants with acute care is 0.46 m/s and the mean speed of participants without is 0.74 m/s
Investigation into the reliability and validity of the measurement of elderly people's clinical walking speed: a systematic review [148] (2012)	86 articles	/	/	Usual and maximum paces are valid tests – usual pace is a reliable test

After a year, researchers measured their usual walking speed and classified participants into three groups: stable (change of gait speed lower than 0.10 m/s), decrease, and increase. Out of all the participants, 18 individuals experienced decreased gait speed, 43 experienced stable gait speed, and ten experienced increased gait speed. The participants whose speed declined had the highest walking speed at baseline and the best results at a narrow walk and stepping over an obstacle. Simple and complex walking while talking was not effective in differentiating the three groups. However, limitations of the study include the small sample size and the lack of consideration for regression potential, even though the fastest at baseline decreased and the slowest at baseline increased. However, a higher gait speed decline appears to be associated with an increase in disabilities, as shown by Artaud et al., which evaluated the association between fast gait speed at baseline, the decline of speed in time, and general disability [152]. Researchers measured the gait speed of 3814 participants from the Three-City Study[43] with two photoelectric cells linked to a stopwatch, as shown in Table 4.1. Individuals were instructed to walk 6 meters several times at their usual and at a fast pace. Disabilities of mobility, instrumental activities of daily living, and basic activities of daily living were reported by the participants during the 11-year follow-up. The mean fast walking speed at baseline was 1.54 m/s, the decline was 0.017 m/s/year, and an accelerated decline was associated with a disability, whereas the fast gait speed at baseline was independent.

4.2. Gait Analysis for Decline of Cognitive Function and Dementia

Dementia and cognitive decline pose a significant burden on the well-being of older populations. Conditions such as Alzheimer's and Parkinson's are associated with significant impairments in movement, thought, and speech, contributing to dementia and affecting the ability of individuals to adequately perform activities of daily living and participate in the social life of their community [153]. There are different types of dementia, such as dementia with Lewy bodies or vascular dementia; these are often difficult to distinguish because of their similarities to other forms of dementia in clinical symptoms [154]. Since many diseases associated with dementia or cognitive decline are conditions that gradually progress and develop over the course of many years, there may be merit for clinicians to be able to perform early detection, as this might allow for interventions to slow down the development of these conditions. This section will discuss existing research pointing to a probable association between gait parameters and a decrease in cognitive function, as well as the potential utility of gait monitoring as a predictive tool in cognitive pathogenesis.

---

[43] A longitudinal study on possible relations between vascular disease and dementia that was conducted in the French cities of Bordeaux, Dijon, and Montpellier.

The association between slow baseline gait speed, change in gait speed, and the hazard of an incident in dementia was assessed by Dumurgier et al. [155]. 3663 participants from the Three-City French prospective cohort were followed up for nine years. Gait speed was measured with two photoelectric cells that were placed 6 meters apart and connected to a chronometer. Participants started the walk 3 meters before the first photoelectric cell and were allowed to keep their usual walking aids, as shown in Table 4.2. Measures were taken at four different times in the project: at baseline, after four years, after seven years, and after nine years. A 0.204 m/s decrease in gait speed (corresponding with 1 - standard deviation) was associated with an increased risk of dementia. This association was relevant for four years and seven years before dementia onset, with a more important hazard ratio for the four years. This means that gait speed begins to slow down approximately seven years before the onset of clinical symptoms of dementia. Furthermore, a longitudinal cohort study of 204 healthy seniors from the Oregon Brain Aging Study established that a significant decrease in gait speed occurs 12.1 years before the clinical symptom of Mild Cognitive Impairment[44] (MCI) [156]. Gait speed was assessed when the participants were walking at their usual speed for 30 feet (9.14 meters), and the interviewer measured time with a stopwatch. During the 20 years of follow-up, gait speed and cognitive function were evaluated each year. A decrease in gait speed that accelerates by 0.023 m/s/y was shown to be a predictor of MCI 12.1 years before the onset.

As demonstrated in studies [155] and [157], assessing the decline of gait speed can be used to predict the development of dementia or MCI. Multiple other studies have confirmed this association, as Quan et al. investigated the association of walking pace with the risk of cognitive decline and dementia by analyzing 17 studies with a reported relative risk and the corresponding 95% confidence interval[45] of cognitive decline and dementia associated with walking pace [158]. Ten studies had values for cognitive decline, and ten studies had values for dementia. By comparing the lowest and highest categories of walking pace, researchers established that the mean relative risk for cognitive decline was 1.89 and the one for dementia was 1.66. Also, every 0.1 m/s decrease in walking pace was associated with a 13% increased risk of dementia, as shown in Table 4.2.

Moreover, another literary review from 2016 highlights the strong association between gait and cognition, as shown in Table 4.2 [159].

---

[44] An intermediate stage between normal cognitive decline associated with aging and serious cognitive decline associated with dementia.

[45] A range of possible values accounting for uncertainty with respect to estimates of the mean.

Researchers have analyzed 50 publications related to cognitive function and gait and have confirmed the hypothesis that gait could be a marker of cognitive decline. They established a hypothesis on how cognition and gait were related to time, suggesting that gait may be a surrogate marker of cognitive decline.

Another study explained the result of a 5-year follow-up of 154 community-dwelling participants aged 65 and older to better determine the association between gait and cognitive function [160]. Gait was tested with the GAITRite® electronic walkway, on which participants had to walk 6 meters, starting and ending 1 meter away from the extremities, to avoid recording the acceleration and deceleration. Cognitive function was tested with the Mini-Mental State Examination (MMSE)[46] and the Montreal Cognitive Assessment[47] (MoCA), which are easy and efficient tests to establish the cognitive function of participants. After a Cox regression and adjustment with a time-dependent covariate, the hazard ratio[48] of the risk of dementia for those with a gait velocity decline was 6.89; 3.61 for those with a cognitive decline; and 7.83 for those with both, suggesting that decline in gait velocity is a better predictor than cognitive decline. They also estimated that the hazard ratio was 1.16 for slow gait at baseline, suggesting that slow gait at baseline is not a good predictor.

For the association between a decline in gait speed and dementia, a study was published in 2018 with a sample of 3932 adults over 60 years old, in which walking speed was measured with a stopwatch and associated with an analysis of the cognitive function, as shown in Table 4.2 [161]. The conclusion was that slower walking speed and greater decline increased the risk of developing dementia. The decrease in walking speed over two years could be an indicator of greater dementia risk. Moreover, the comparison with the result of the cognitive test demonstrates that walking speed and cognitive capacity can predict dementia independently.

In compliance with the previously mentioned study [161], slow gait speed is a good predictor of cognitive decline, as also elucidated by Mielke et al. in a study which included 1478 cognitively normal participants who were evaluated every 15 months with a nurse visit, neurologic evaluation, and neuropsychological testing [162]. Moreover, timed gait speed was assessed over 25 feet (7.6 meters), and the study aimed to conduct a temporal analysis

---

[46] A short questionnaire assessing various areas of cognitive function, including attention, recall, and language.
[47] A cognitive screening test that assists health professionals in identifying possible cognitive impairment or indicators of Alzheimer's disease.
[48] Ratio of event probabilities with risk exposure relative to baseline probabilities.

of the association between cognitive functions and gait speed. Faster gait speed was associated with better performance in memory, executive function, and global cognition. Faster gait speed at baseline was associated with less cognitive decline across the all-domain specific and global scores. By contrast, baseline cognition was not associated with changes in gait speed. Thus, a slow gait precedes cognitive decline.

In addition, a longitudinal aging cohorts' study has established that walking speed was particularly correlated with modifications in fluid cognition by studying 36 publications concerning the cognitive and executive functions of which walking speed was a parameter [163]. Fluid cognition is a part of cognition related to the maintenance of information and memory [164]. The research compared different executive functions (e.g., grip strength and flamingo stand time) and different cognitive functions (e.g., mental state and fluid cognition), where the main goal was to find executive parameters and their corresponding cognitive functions.

Furthermore, another study evaluated the relative contributions of specific elements of cognitive function to dual-task gait speed in a nationally representative population of 4431 community-dwelling adults over 50 years old in Ireland [165]. For this purpose, gait speed was obtained using the GAITRite® walkway during three gait tasks: single, cognitive (alternate letters), and motor (carrying a filled glass). Linear regression models adjusted for covariates were constructed to observe the differences brought about in gait speed by seven different neuropsychological tests. This study was also used to outline other effects on gait that were brought about by tasks. For the cohort that was observed in this study, the results established a direct and independent association between gait speed and gait tasks. Dual gait tasks highlighted specific elements of the brain's executive function.

A Japanese study has demonstrated that low trajectories for gait speed and step length were significantly associated with incident-disabling dementia [166]. They assessed the step length and gait speed of 1686 adults, without dementia, aged between 65 and 90, with an 11-meter walkway. The participants were instructed to walk at their usual and maximum pace while the staff measured the time needed to walk 5 meters. The development of dementia was evaluated with Japanese long-term care insurance data. Three distinct trajectory patterns (high, middle, and low) based on their gait speeds and step lengths were identified, and with adjusting results, the study demonstrated that the individuals from the low group were 3.46 times as likely to develop dementia than the higher group.

The association between balance, gait parameters, and decline in cognitive function for post-stroke patients was investigated in a 2015 study [167]. Walking parameters of 298 patients with mild-moderate ischemic stroke or transient ischemic attack from the Tel Aviv Brain Acute Stroke Cohort study were measured with a stopwatch, and their cognitive functions were evaluated during the 2-year follow-up, as shown in Table 4.2. Cognitive decline was highly associated with a poorer result on the TUG test, lower Berg Balance Scale scores, and slower gait speed. Thus, gait speed was found to be a good predictor of cognitive decline in the two years after stroke.

Another study analyzed a French prospective cohort and aimed to determine the association between gait speed, psychomotor speed, and incident dementia [155]. The gait speed and cognitive capacity of 1265 participants over 65 years of age were measured at baseline, and the incidence of dementia was determined over the 12-year follow-up period. The gait speed assessment was a 3-meter walk and back at their usual walking speed, and the time to cover the 6-meter distance was measured by the interviewer. Both gait speed and psychomotor speed were concluded to be independent predictors of all-cause dementia and Alzheimer's disease.

A publication related to Alzheimer's disease (AD) was published in 2018 [168]. Fourteen patients with AD and the same number without AD were instructed to take walking tests during which the time to walk a 6-meter straight and a 6-meter curved path was measured with a stopwatch, as shown in Table 4.2. Measures on global cognition were also realized, and it was shown that participants with AD had a significantly slower gait than the healthy group for a straight and curved path.

Slow gait speed and decline in gait speed are not the only parameters that could be used to predict cognitive decline, as demonstrated in a study which found associations between a specific cognitive function and a specific parameter [169]. Velocity, cadence, and a coefficient of variance in stride length were assessed in single- and dual-task conditions with the GAITRite® system for 671 participants from the Einstein Aging Study. The cognitive function evaluated the domains of Executive Attention, Verbal IQ, and Memory. After a linear regression, it was established that executive attention is associated with velocity in single and dual conditions and the coefficient of variance in stride length. Memory is related to velocity and cadence in both walking conditions. Thus, the association between cognitive function and gait walking depends on the gait parameters and the walking condition.

The relationship between quantitative gait parameters, a decline in specific cognitive domains, and the risk of developing dementia was examined by Verghese et al. [4]. To this end, researchers conducted a prospective cohort study with 427 participants aged 70 years and older, of whom 399 were dementia-free and were followed up for five years. In the beginning, their quantitative gait parameters, representing pace, rhythm, and variability, were measured with embedded pressure gait sensors. An increase in the rhythm factor was associated with a more important memory decline. On the contrary, the pace factor was associated with a decline in executive function. With Cox models adjusted for age, sex, and education, an increase in baseline rhythm and variability factor scores was associated with an increased risk of dementia. The pace factor predicted the risk of developing vascular dementia with a hazard ratio of 1.60. The study did not analyze every possible aspect of gait; however, most of the gait parameters that were not measured are derived from or highly correlated with the selected ones.

A study conducted with 2332 participants from the population-based Swedish National Study on Aging and Care in Kungsholmen, Sweden, assessed the relationship between walking speed, processing speed, changes in walking and processing speed, and dementia [170]. Walking speed was calculated as the time taken to cover 2.4 meters or 6 meters at a chosen speed measured by the nurses. The apparition of dementia was diagnosed during the six years after baseline. Without adjustment for processing speed, the participants with a slow baseline walking speed and those with a decline in their walking speed over time had a higher risk of dementia, with a respective odds ratio of 1.61 and 2.58. The cross-parameter results showed that the participants with good performance at walking speed and poor performance at processing speed were those who developed dementia.

Another study with 811 adults aged older than 65 from the Baltimore Longitudinal Study of Aging used data on the 400-meter walk test and calculated the variation of the lap time with ten 40-meter laps [171]. Researchers also collected the usual speed of the participants by measuring the time they took to walk 6 meters and measuring their cognitive functions with different tests. After statistical tests, they concluded that an important variation in lap time was associated with psychomotor slowing at all speeds and that for fast walkers, an important variation was associated with worse cognitive flexibility. Later, the same researchers conducted another study evaluating the relationship between baseline lap time variation and longitudinal change in executive function [172]. In this study, they used the same 400-meter walk test on 347 participants and assessed their executive function with different tests, including attention, cognitive flexibility and set-shifting, visuo-perceptual speed, and working memory. They concluded that higher lap time variability was only a predictor of a decline in performance for cognitive flexibility and set-shifting.

A British structured review studied the differences in gait characteristics between healthy controls and four subtypes of dementia: dementia with Lewy bodies, vascular dementia, Alzheimer's disease, and Parkinson's disease dementia [173]. They analyzed 26 papers in which dementia was associated with gait characteristics by a slower pace, impaired rhythm, and increased variability. Contrary to expectations, participants in the subtype of Alzheimer's disease dementia were less impaired in pace, rhythm, and variability domains of gait than the other dementias. Of the 26 studies, only four were comparing different types of dementia; thus, more studies are needed to establish a more prominent association of gait to differentiate different types of dementia.

A study conducted between 2002 and 2015 to assess the validity of dementia prediction with the walking-while-talking test was published in 2018 [174]. The study sample was composed of 1156 older adults from the Einstein Aging Study. The gait parameters were measured with the GAITRite® system over a distance of 180 inches (4.5 meters), with the acceleration and deceleration phases eliminated. Variability and step time standard derivation were shown to be predictors of incident dementia (hazard ratio = 1.24) and vascular dementia (hazard ratio = 1.50). However, variability and swing time standard derivation were not significantly associated with the risk of incident Alzheimer's disease and dementia.

To predict the risks of developing dementia on a daily basis, a study was conducted to design a system for the task [175]. Researchers analyzed the gait of 74 older adults with a 24 GHz micro-Doppler radar and assessed their cognitive capacity with different tests (e.g., verbal fluency test). After statistical analysis, they were able to conclude that the walking parameters were effective in classifying older adults with lower cognitive functions. They also determined that all cognitive functions have a better statistical association with the leg velocity in the swing phase than with the walking speed. Finally, the different gait velocity parameters were associated with each cognitive domain, meaning that the walking observation could be used to determine which cognitive domain was impacted. However, the limitations of this study include a small number of participants and a limitation of analysis to a few cognitive domains.

Table 4.2. Gait analysis for decline of cognitive function and dementia

Study	Sample	Method of Analysis	Duration of the follow-up	Conclusion
Quantitative gait dysfunction and risk of cognitive decline and dementia [4] (2007)	427 adults over 70 of which 28 had dementia	Embedded pressure gait sensors	5 years	Increase on baseline rhythm and variability factor scores is associated with higher risk of dementia {hazard ratio} = 1.60
The trajectory of gait speed preceding mild cognitive impairment [156] (2010)	204 healthy seniors	Stopwatch (30-feet)	20 years	A decline of 0.023 m/s/year can be a predictor of Mild Cognitive Impairment 12.1 years before the clinical symptom
Assessing the temporal relationship between cognition and gait: slow gait predicts cognitive decline in the Mayo Clinic Study of Aging [162] (2013)	1478 participants	Stopwatch (25-feet)	4.1 years	Faster gait speed at baseline is associated with better global cognition and baseline cognition is not associated with changes in gait speed
The dynamic relationship between physical function and cognition in longitudinal aging cohorts [163] (2013)	36 studies (literary review)	/	/	Walk speed is highly correlated to variation in fluid cognition (related with memory)
Walking speed, processing speed, and dementia: a population-based longitudinal study [170] (2014)	2332 participants	Stopwatch (6 meters or 2.4 meters)	6 years	Processing speed might be a better predictor of dementia than walking speed
Relative association of processing speed, short-term memory and sustained attention with task on gait speed: A study of community-dwelling people 50 years and older [165] (2014)	4431 participants (mean age = 62.4 years)	GAITRite® walkway during three gait tasks: single, cognitive (alternate letters), and motor (carrying a filled glass)	/	Participants with poorer processing speed, short-term memory and sustained attention walked more slowly at baseline for single and dual task

Study	Sample	Method of Analysis	Duration of the follow-up	Conclusion
The relationship between attention and gait in aging: Facts and fallacies [169] (2012)	671 participants	GAITRite® system	/	The association between cognitive function and gait walking depends on the gait parameters and the walking condition
Lap time variation and executive function in older adults: The Baltimore Longitudinal Study of Aging [171] (2015)	811 adults older than 65 years	Stopwatch (400 meter with laps of 40 meters)	/	An important lap time variation was associated with a psychomotor slowing for all speed and that for fast walker, an important variation was associated with worse cognitive flexibility
Intra-individual lap time variation of the 400-m walk, an early mobility indicator of executive function decline in high-functioning older adults? [172] (2015)	347 adults aged 60 and older	Stopwatch (400 meter with laps of 40 meters)	/	Lap time variability is a predictor of decline in performance for cognitive flexibility and set shifting
Gait and cognition: mapping the global and discrete relationships in ageing and neurodegenerative disease [159] (2016)	50 publications (literary review)	/	/	There is a strong association between gait speed and cognition. Gait speed can predict cognition decline
Gait performance trajectories and incident disabling dementia among community-dwelling older Japanese [166] (2017)	1686 adults aged 65 to 90	Stopwatch (11 meters)	12 years	Low group were 3.46 times higher risk to develop dementia than the fast group
Walking pace and the risk of cognitive decline and dementia in elderly populations: a meta-analysis of prospective cohort studies [158] (2017)	17 studies (literary review) with 9,949 participants for cognitive risk and 14,140 for dementia	/	/	The relative risk for comparing the lowest and the highest category of walking pace for cognitive decline was 1.89 and the one for dementia was 1.66. Every 0.1 m/s decrement in walking pace was associated with a 13% increased risk of dementia.

Table 4.2. (Continued)

Study	Sample	Method of Analysis	Duration of the follow-up	Conclusion
Gait speed and decline in gait speed as predictors of incident dementia [155] (2017)	3,663 participants (mean age = 73.5 years)	Two photoelectric cells placed 6 meters apart and connected to a chronometer	9 years	A 0.204 m/s lower gait speed is associated with increase of hazard dementia {hazard ratio} = 1.46, 4 years before the onset dementia. Gait is slower up 7 years before the onset dementia
Association of gait speed, psychomotor speed, and dementia [157] (2017)	1,265 adults over 65 years	Stopwatch (3 meters)	12 years	Gait speed and psychomotor speed were independent predictors of all-cause dementia and Alzheimer's disease
What can quantitative gait analysis tell us about dementia and its subtypes? A structured review [173] (2017)	26 papers about gait speed and subtypes of dementia	/	/	Alzheimer's diseases are less impaired in pace, rhythm and variability domains of gait than the other dementias
Walking while talking and risk of incident dementia [174] (2018)	1156 elderly individuals (mean age: 78.28 years)	GAITRite® system over a distance of 180 inches (4.5 meters)	Median follow-up of 1.90 years old	Variability and step time standard derivation are predictor of incident dementia ({hazard ratio} = 1.24) and vascular dementia ({hazard ratio} = 1.50)
Walking speed, cognitive function, and dementia risk in the English Longitudinal Study of Ageing [161] (2018)	3932 individuals aged 60 and older	Stopwatch (8-feet walk)	Follow-up every 2 years from 2002 to 2015	Slower walking speed and greater decline increased the risk of dementia. Decrease of walking speed is also an indicator of dementia

Study	Sample	Method of Analysis	Duration of the follow-up	Conclusion
Motor and cognitive trajectories before dementia: results from gait and brain study [160] (2018)	154 community-dwelling individuals aged 65 and older	6-meter walk on the GAITRite® electronic system	5 years	{hazard ratio} = 6.89 of dementia for people with a gait velocity decline; {hazard ratio} = 3.61 for those with cognitive decline and {hazard ratio} = 7.83 for those with both
The effect of walking path configuration on gait in adults with Alzheimer's dementia [168] (2018)	14 participants with Alzheimer's diseases and 14 without	Stopwatch	/	AD patient are significantly slower walkers than healthy people
Gait measures as predictors of poststroke cognitive function: Evidence from the TABASCO Study [167] (2015)	298 participants were patients with first-ever, mild-moderate ischemic stroke or transient ischemic attack		2 years	The results of this study suggest that measures of gait and balance are significant risk markers of cognitive status after 2 years of occurrence of stroke
Using micro-doppler radar to measure gait features associated with cognitive functions in elderly adults [175] (2019)	74 elderly adults over 75 years	24 GHz micro-Doppler radar	/	Walking parameters are effective to detect individuals with lower cognitive function and that leg velocity in the swing phase was a better predictor than gait speed

4.3. Gait Analysis and Central Nervous System

As evidenced in Table 4.2, there appears to be an association between gait speed and cognitive function. However, brain physiology alone is not sufficient in explaining the connection between cognitive decline and changes in motor functions such as walking because body-wide movement is fundamentally a product of the brain's ability to integrate its function with various parts of the nervous network outside the skull area. Therefore, no discussion on the link between gait and cognitive function is complete without considering the essential role of both the peripheral and central nervous systems.

Cognition and motor functions are functionally connected, as both are controlled by various parts of the brain, such as the frontal lobes, cerebellum, hippocampus, and basal ganglia [176]. However, it is the wider nervous system (NS) that must be holistically considered when evaluating the true impact of cognitive decline on gait function. The central nervous system (CNS) is a complex system composed of the brain and the spinal cord. It is referred to as "central" because it combines information from the entire body and coordinates activity in the organism.

The anatomy of the brain can be divided into the brain's hemisphere, the cerebellum, the diencephalon (thalamus, hypothalamus, and epithalamus), the hippocampus, and the brain stem. Each part has white matter and grey matter: the white matter's role is to connect different parts of the grey matter. The brain has different areas (frontal lobe, occipital lobe, parietal lobe, and temporal lobe) that control different functions of the body (e.g., the motor areas are in the back of the frontal lobe). The basal ganglia and grey matter of the brain are essential in controlling motor activity in the body, such as control and movement execution.

The spinal cord, the second essential part of the nervous system, spans the back of the human body and carries information between the brain and the body while simultaneously performing other tasks. Along the length, it connects with the nerves of the peripheral nervous system (PNS) that run in the skin, muscles, and joints. The consciously controlled or "voluntary" component of the PNS is known as the somatic nervous system and consists of sensory and motor neurons. Sensory neurons originate in tissues such as the skin and carry "input" information that is relayed to the brain and spinal cord. The CNS then directs signals that travel along motor neurons that control skeletal muscles, producing bodily movement. There are circuits within the spine that control reflexive movements, such as withdrawing the hand when it

Pathological Implications of Gait 63

comes into contact with a threatening stimulus (e.g., flames). Similar circuits in the spine are also equipped to control more complex movements, such as walking.

Interestingly, movements such as walking depend more critically on the spinal cord than the brain. In an experiment, the brain of the cat was separated from the spinal cord, and the cat could still walk, which suggested that the role of the brain is essentially to start and stop movement, whereas the spinal cord is more responsible for carrying forward the actual movement as it can coordinate all muscle movements necessary to walk [177]. Table 4.3 summarizes key findings from various studies on gait abnormalities associated with neurological disorders, highlighting the impact of central nervous system dysfunction on walking patterns and motor control.

A publication reported key findings from the conference of the Gerontological Society of America in collaboration with the National Institute on Aging and the University of Pittsburgh regarding the association between aging, speed of gait, and the central nervous system [178]. The data concerning gait came from a database that used force-sensitive switches to measure the gait of participants. The main conclusion was that the CNS was an important contributor to mobility limitations, even for people without any visible cognitive trouble. Another study established a longitudinal association between gait parameters and white or grey matter lesions [179]. The volume and the potential presence of lesions in the white matter, the hippocampi, and the grey matter were analyzed with MRI. Walking was measured with GAITRite®, and each patient was instructed to walk a 4.6-meter distance six times. Gait variables such as speed, component cadence, step length, and step width were calculated over the six walks. The mean follow-up was 30.6 months, and the study concluded that white matter atrophy, white matter lesions, hippocampal atrophy, and total gray matter atrophy were associated with the decline of at least one of the gait parameters. In a different study, other gait parameters were measured with the GAITRite® system, and White Matter Lesions (WMLs) were measured with MRI for 294 individuals [180]. The study showed that the increased size and volume of the lesions were associated with an increase in gait variability and a decrease in gait quality. A literature review conducted by researchers from the Health Sciences Research and Neurology Department of the Mayo Clinic in Rochester, USA, summarized the studies investigating the association between gait, neuropathologies, and the different parts of the brain [181]. Grey matter atrophy was found to be most associated with poorer gait performance. Moreover, by comparing different research studies, the researchers established that both hyper and hypo actions were linked with gait modification. Finally, there are some early pieces of evidence that amyloid and tau protein aggregation harm gait parameters. The review highlights the fact that, while there is a lack of information about the association between brain areas and gait parameters, some of the existing information in the literature is promising.

Another study investigates the importance of β-amyloid in gait modification and neurological diseases [182]. The association between brain β-amyloid and gait speed for 128 older adult patients from a pool of healthy controls to mildly cognitively impaired patients was studied. Gait speed was defined as the time needed for the participant to cover a walkway of 4 meters. The brain β-amyloid measures were obtained via a semiautomated quantitative analysis using the cerebellum as a reference region. An association was found between slow gait speed and β-amyloid in different parts of the brain: the posterior and anterior putamen, the occipital cortex, the precuneus, and the anterior cingulate. β-amyloid was responsible for 9% of the variance in gait speed. Moreover, β-amyloid, via neurofibrillary tangles and plaques that accumulate as the result of a gene mutation that causes dysfunctional protein splicing, is implicated in the development of Alzheimer's disease (AD). This study thus establishes a possible relationship between AD and motor function.

An analysis of the variability of the step length, the variability of the stance time, and the variability of the step width was performed using an electronic walkway system on 558 participants from the Pittsburgh site of the Cardiovascular Health Study [183]. Researchers also analyzed the participants' impairments, including central nervous system function, sensory function, and strength. They found an association between central nervous system impairment and stance time variability, especially for slow walkers. Sensory impairments had an impact on step width variability for fast walkers.

The "motoric cognitive risk" (MCR) syndrome is a predementia syndrome combining cognitive complaints and slow gait speed. A study from the Gerontological Society of America aimed to compare the cognitive profile of nondemented older community dwellers with and without MCR syndrome and to examine the association of global and regional brain volumes with MCR syndrome [184]. They measured different parts of the brain in 171 individuals (28 MCR and 143 non-MCR) by MRI. Other parameters, such as age, the number of drugs taken daily, and cognitive profile, were also measured. Gait speed was assessed with a GAITRite® system. The results showed that the cognitive profile was the same for MCR and non-MCR patients; however, MCR-related smaller global and regional grey matter volumes involving premotor and prefrontal cortices suggested that the MCR syndrome may predict cortical neurodegenerative dementia more than subcortical dementia. In addition, Allali et al. defined different subtypes of MCR according to which gait parameter was the most impacted; cognitive complaint was still a factor of MCR for all subtypes [185]. MCRv represented slow gait velocity, MCRsl represented short stride length, MCRsw represented slow swing time, and MCRslv represented high stride length variability. These subtypes were not mutually exclusive. Researchers analyzed the cognitive function of 314 patients diagnosed with MCR. The patient's gait was measured with a GAITRite® system. Out of all the participants, 84.7% did not meet the criteria for any of the subtypes, but the analysis of those who did shows that MCRv was associated with deficits in attention and language, thus suggesting that incident cognitive impairment in global conditions and MCRsw were associated with deficits in all cognitive domains, including memory.

Neurodegenerative diseases (NDDs), like Parkinson's disease, are pathologies that affect the brain and sometimes the gait as well. Parkinson's, for instance, is associated with a loss of neurons facilitating the transmission of dopamine, which plays a major role in regulating motor control. Associations between the gait and the NDDs could be a way to understand the association between gait and CNS if the NDDs studied are well known. For example, there is already some evidence that stride-to-stride variations in gait cycle timing depend on basal ganglia function [186]. In the study, gait analysis was conducted to investigate the stride-to-stride variation of gait cycle timing in patients with NDDs. Researchers measured the gait parameters of 15 patients with Parkinson's disease (PD), 20 patients with Huntington's disease (HD), and 16 healthy controls with force-resistive sensors. Each measure of gait variability was two to three times increased for PD and HD patients compared to healthy patients, and the degree of gait variability was correlated with disease severity. This hypothesis has been confirmed and has assessed the reliability of gait variability for patients with Parkinson's disease [187]. Researchers asked 27 older individuals and 25 PD participants to walk continuously for two minutes and to do three intermittent walks over a 12-meter walkway. Gait characteristics were assessed with the GAITRite® electronic mat, and gait variability was calculated based on step velocity, length and width, step, stance, and swing duration. They established that gait variability was more reliable during continuous walks than intermittent walks and that the most reliable protocol to predict Parkinson's disease was a 30-step continuous walk.

The relationship between walking speed and gait variability for patients with Parkinson's disease and healthy controls was evaluated in a 2005 study [188]. It was already known that PD patients have a gait rhythm impairment, which can be quantified by measuring the variability of gait timing in stride-to-stride. Researchers used a treadmill to assess the gait parameters of 36 patients with PD and 30 healthy controls. The treadmill was used at four different speeds: comfortable walking speed (CWS), as well as 80%, 90%, and 110% of the CWS. A 10-meter walking test was also conducted with a stopwatch. The research confirmed that the variability of stride and swing is higher for PD patients than for healthy controls. Also, at the range studied, swing time variability is independent of gait speed and can be used as a marker of rhythmicity. Finally, stride time variability and swing time variability are not both affected in the same way by gait speed, meaning that these two parameters are not controlled by the same brain mechanism. Moreover, an Italian study established that Parkinson's disease patients with mild cognitive impairment (MCI) have a reduced step length, a reduced swing time, and a diminution of stability [189]. Researchers also demonstrated that visuospatial impairments were associated with instability, particularly for PD patients. They measured the gait parameters of 19 patients with PD and MCI, 24 patients with PD but without MCI, and 20 healthy participants with an optokinetic system (with a set of six infrared cameras, a ProReflex Motion Capture Unit, and data acquisition software). Participants were assessed with three walking tests: normal gait, motor dual-task, and cognitive dual-task. Step length, swing time, and stability were shown to be reduced for participants with PD and MCI, particularly with a dual task.

Some researchers have already proven that gait dynamics could help diagnose NDDs [190]. Data from another study was used to create a training set for deterministic learning [183]. The conclusion was that deterministic learning was effective in separating the gait patterns of healthy participants and patients with NDDs [191]. Another recent study used the same data to lead a statistical analysis of the gait parameters in NDDs [192]. Researchers studied swing, stance, stride, and double support intervals for healthy participants and patients with NDDs. They were also able to differentiate the different pathologies of NDDs; thus, a statistical analysis of gait parameters could also help diagnose NDDs.

Table 4.3. Gait analysis and central nervous system

Study	Sample	Method of Analysis	Duration of the Follow-up	Conclusion
Gait variability and basal ganglia disorders: stride-to-stride variations of gait cycle timing in Parkinson's disease and Huntington's disease [186] (1998)	16 healthy controls, 15 patients with Parkinson's disease and 20 patients with Huntington's disease	Force-sensitive resistors measuring a 5-minute walk	/	PD and HD were associated with an increase of the variability of the gait parameters
Effect of gait speed on gait rhythmicity in Parkinson's disease: variability of stride time and swing time respond differently [188] (2005)	36 patients with PD and 30 healthy participants	Treadmill and 10-meter walk measured with a stopwatch	/	Swing time variability is independent of gait speed. Gait speed doesn't impact stride time and swing time variability the same way meaning that these parameters are not controlled by the same mechanism
Gait patterns in Parkinsonian patients with or without mild cognitive impairment [189] (2012)	19 patients with PD and mild cognitive impairment, 24 with PD and without MCI and 20 healthy patients	Optokinetic system (with a set of 6 infrared cameras, a ProReflex Motion Capture Unit and data acquisition software	/	Parkinson's disease patients with mild cognitive impairment (MCI) had reduced step length, reduced swing time and diminution of stability. Visuospatial impairment was associated with instability
Is gait variability reliable in older adults and Parkinson's disease? Towards an optimal testing protocol [187] (2013)	27 older adults and 25 Parkinson's disease patient	GAITRite® electronic walkway	/	The most reliable protocol to predict Parkinson's diseases is a 30-step continuous walk

Table 4.3. (Continued)

Study	Sample	Method of Analysis	Duration of the Follow-up	Conclusion
Classification of neurodegenerative diseases using gait dynamics via deterministic learning [190] (2015)	16 healthy controls, 48 patients with three different neurodegenerative diseases (NDDs)	Force-sensitive resistors and derivation of the data obtained	/	Deterministic learning of gait can help diagnose NDDs
Comprehensive statistical analysis of the gait parameters in neurodegenerative diseases [192] (2018)	16 healthy controls, 46 patients with three different neurodegenerative diseases (NDDs)	Force-sensitive resistors and derivation of the data obtained	/	Statistical analysis of gait parameters can differentiate the types of NDDs
Aging, the central nervous system, and mobility [178] (2013)	Workshop (75 scientists)	Force-sensitive switches	/	CNS is an important contributor to mobility limitations in older adults without overt neurological disease
Brain structural change and gait decline: a longitudinal population-based study [179] (2013)	225 participants aged between 60 and 86	GAITRite®	30.6 months	Gait speed is impacted by white matter lesions, atrophy, hippocampal atrophy and grey matter atrophy
Cerebral white matter lesions, gait, and the risk of incident falls a prospective population-based study [180] (2009)	294 participants (mean age 72.3 years), independently mobile	GAITRite®	/	White matter lesions are strong risk factors for falls in the general older population
Association between various brain pathologies and gait disturbance [181] (2017)	Literary review (31 studies)		14 years	All pathologies reviewed were associated with gait, grey matter atrophy was most consistently linked with poorer gait performance.
Relationship of regional brain β-amyloid to gait speed [182] (2016)	128 participants		/	Association was concluded between Alzheimer's disease pathology and impacted gait speed

Study	Sample	Method of Analysis	Duration of the Follow-up	Conclusion
Stance time and step width variability have unique contributing impairments in older persons [183] (2008)	558 participants	Computerized walkway	/	Increased stance time variability is associated with increased CNS impairment while decreased step width variability is associated with increased sensory impairment
Association of motoric cognitive risk syndrome with brain volumes: results from the GAIT Study [184] (2016)	171 individuals (28 MCR and 143 non-MCR)	GAITRite® system	/	MCR syndrome is associated with slower gait speed
Motoric cognitive risk syndrome subtypes and cognitive profiles [185] (2015)	314 participants 65 and older, diagnosed with MCR but non-demented	Walkway with embedded pressure sensors	728 days	MCR subtypes based on individual gait parameters show commonalities and differences in cognitive profiles and risk factors
Altered fractal dynamics of gait: reduced stride-interval correlations with aging and Huntington's disease. [193] (1997)	10 subjects from Harvard database 70 years or older with excellent health with no previous history of falls and 17 subjects with Huntington's disease who could walk for five minutes	Force sensitive switches	/	Stride-interval correlations are decreased with advanced age and with HD and are probably dependent on intact central nervous system processing but are independent of walking speed and variability

4.4. Gait Analysis and Fall Prediction

Falls are a very common injury among older adults and are linked to wider changes in cognitive and motor function as individuals age. They occur in a wide variety of environments but are very commonly associated with homes and nursing care facilities, in which the often inadequately ergonomic design of inhabited spaces (e.g., beds, staircases, etc.) frequently poses risks to the safety of older adults [194]. Falls, which often result in conditions of physical trauma such as hip fractures, are a constraining injury with potentially severe implications for the ability of individuals to perform activities of daily living. They are a major source of hospitalization among older adults and exert a steep yet preventable toll on clinical resources that can potentially be diverted to more pressing and complex health issues. Should gait monitoring be identified as an effective mechanism for predicting falls, this would represent a significant victory for the cause of senior health overall.

Gait speed also seems to be related to fall prediction, as demonstrated by Quach et al., which analyzed data from 763 community-dwelling older adults, of whom 600 were followed up for 18 months, as shown in Table 4.4 [195]. An interviewer measured the time taken to walk a 4-meter distance with a stopwatch, which was then used to calculate gait speed. Researchers collected information about the fall with monthly postcard calendars and differentiated indoor and outdoor falls. There was a U-shaped relationship between gait speed and falls: slow walkers had the highest risk of falling indoors, while fast walkers had the highest risk of falling outdoors. Those with the lowest risk of falling were the normal speed walkers, whose speed is between 1.0 m/s and 1.3 m/s [195]. One of the most useful pieces of information about gait for predicting pathologies is the reduction of speed with time. Thus, it is necessary to regularly measure gait speed. Another study compared an average in-home speed (AIGS) to a set of traditional physical performance instruments (habitual gait speed, TUG, short physical performance battery, Berg Balance Scale (short form), and Multidirectional Reach Test) used for mobility and fall risk assessment of older adults, as shown in Table 4.4 [196]. AIGS appeared to demonstrate the best performance, given that it measured everyday walking.

However, slow gait speed seems to be neither unique nor the best predictor of falls. Indeed, it was demonstrated that the gait variables related to a higher risk of falls for cerebellar ataxia patients were slow gait speed and temporal gait variability [197]. Cerebellar ataxia is a pathology resulting from the inflammation of the cerebellum that generally causes loss of coordination, difficulty walking, and hence, falls. Researchers used a 6.7-meter GAITRite®

electronic walkway to analyze the gait parameters of 48 patients with eight different types of cerebellar ataxia. Fall events were categorized, and gait variability in the fore-aft direction was used to show the difference between the groups. The most relevant parameters associated with the fall risk for patients with cerebellar ataxia were slow walking and temporal gait variability; the accuracy of fall prediction was increased using speed-dependent integrals of gait variability, as shown in Table 4.4.

Researchers from the University of Hull in the United Kingdom assessed whether there was an association between gait parameters, walking speed, and bone mineral density (BMD) for older postmenopausal women [198]. BMD is known to be related to falls. The gait speed of 45 post-menopausal women was measured with 12 motion capture cameras sampling at 100 Hz. The mean walking speed was 1.40 m/s; according to the researchers, this measure explained most of the variance in the gait parameters. Moreover, the speed associated with the T-score[49] explained some of the knee joint variables [198].

A team of researchers who previously established a relationship between gait parameters and cognitive function [4] conducted a study to identify quantitative gait markers of falls [199]. They used a computerized walkway with embedded pressure sensors to analyze the gait of 597 adults aged 70 or older. The parameters studied were speed, cadence, stride length, swing, double support, stride length variability, and swing time variability. The association of these parameters with the incident fall rate was studied using generalized estimation equation procedures adjusted for age, sex, education, falls, chronic illnesses, medications, cognition, disability, and traditional clinical tests of gait and balance. Slower gait speed was associated with a higher risk of falls in the fully adjusted models. Among six other markers, participants who had the worst performance on the swing double-support phase, swing time variability, and stride length variability fell more than those with a better result. Increased stride length and swing time variability were the most robust predictors of falls and were the only predictors of injurious falls. Studies on dual-task tests (e.g., walking while talking) have shown that while speed was modified in healthy patients, the variability of stride was not, suggesting that the regulation of variability is normally automated and requires minimal cognitive input [200]. Thus, patients with cognitive impairment lose the ability to know how to walk and fall, as shown in Table 4.4.

A study aimed to investigate the association between slow gait speed and fall risks in nursing homes [201]. Researchers measured gait speed as the time

---

[49] A score that establishes the advancement of osteoporosis.

taken to cover a 40-foot (12.19-meter) distance with a chronometer. They also studied the association between falls and other factors, including fear of falling and environmental causes. The sample consisted of 16 participants, out of whom five fell during the 6-month follow-up. This study concluded that gait speed is not linked to falls in nursing homes but that environmental causes are. However, the small sample and the short follow-up are major limitations of the study, as shown in Table 4.4.

Overall, these studies provide support for temporal gait variability, increased stride length, and increased swing time variability as complementary predictors of falls and more reliable predictors of falls than gait speed. Several studies have analyzed the relationship between the risk of falls and the variability of one or multiple gait parameters, one involving 52 community-living ambulatory patients of a geriatric clinic, demonstrating that stride time variability was higher for participants who experienced a fall [20]. The stride time variability was measured with force-sensitive insoles that participants wore while walking for six minutes. Falls were reported weekly for a year after the baseline test. The researchers were able to demonstrate, using logistic regression, that stride time variability predicted falls and that there was a correlation between stride time variability and other factors, such as gait speed or balance. However, the limitations of the study include a small sample size and a short follow-up period.

A linear association between variability in step length, double-support phase, and increased odds of multiple falls was established by Callisaya et al. [194]. The gait speed of 412 participants aged between 60 and 86 years was measured with an electronic walkway (GAITRite® system), and their falls were tracked over the course of a year. The researchers also revealed non-linear associations between gait speed, cadence, step time variability, and the increased risk of multiple falls. There were no factors associated with a single risk of falling, as described in Table 4.4. Local Dynamic Stability (LDS) is a health parameter that can be estimated by measuring gait using, for example, a trunk accelerometer to detect falls [202]. LDS is derived from the chaos theory and evaluates the sensitivity of gait to small perturbations naturally due to internal causes and external disturbances. LDS was calculated as the average exponential rate of deviation among trajectories in a state that reflected the gait dynamics. Eighty-three participants with mild to moderate neurological disorders and 40 healthy controls wore a belt 3-axis accelerometer while walking for at least 30 seconds in a 70-meter hallway. Data analysis revealed that the relative difference in the LDS for patients and healthy controls was 33%, with a greater LDS for patients with neurological disorders that had a higher risk of falls. LDS was reliable in differentiating between individuals with a risk of falling and participants without a risk of falling. The association between gait speed, LDS, and the risk of falling was investigated by Toebes et al. [203]. Gait parameters and LDS of 134 participants were assessed with a worn accelerometer, and fall history was reported during the following year. The conclusion was that gait variability and increased LDS were predictors of falls for older adults.

Multiple sclerosis (MS) is an autoimmune pathology that affects the central nervous system. It involves T-cells breaching the blood-brain barrier and reacting to (i.e., attacking) the myelin. Myelin is important for the efficiency of nerve signal movement and facilitates a process called saltatory conduction in which electrical impulses "skip" from node to node. In the absence of saltatory conduction, the nerve signal would experience a long, drawn-out "dying down" as it traveled along the axon. MS has been associated with a loss of strength, cognitive impairment, and a decrease in coordination. A study evaluated the association between falls in women with MS, balance, gait, and strength [204]. Researchers used an instrumented walkway system to measure the gait parameters of 99 women with MS. They also assessed balance with the limits of the stability test and the Sensory Organization Test. The study revealed a correlation between MS and falls, with a total of 159 falls by 48% of participants within a year. Lack of stability, stand-phase asymmetries, and base-of-support width during gait were identified as likely predictors of falls for women with MS.

Gait analysis to predict falls can be realized with an electronic walkway with embedded sensors, as demonstrated in some previous studies, but it has also been shown that other methods are valid and reliable that demonstrate the possibility of using micro-Doppler radar to detect the fallers [205]. Data was obtained with a 60 GHz micro-Doppler radar, along with velocity parameters, from three subject groups: healthy young and older adults, and older adults with a history of falls were tracked using a motion capture system (Mocap). These findings establish that different walking patterns exist and could be separated by studying walking. However, other studies need to be done to verify the reliability of the experiment.

Table 4.4. Gait analysis and fall prediction

Study	Sample	Method of Analysis	Duration of the Follow-up	Conclusions
Gait variability and fall risk in community-living older adults: a 1-year prospective study [20] (2001)	52 patients of geriatric clinic	Force-sensitive insoles (6-minute walk)	1 year	Stride time variability is higher for participants that experienced falls
Quantitative gait markers and incident fall risk in older adults [199] (2009)	597 adults aged 70 or older	Computerized walkway with embedded pressure sensors	Mean of 20 months	Slower gait speed was associated with higher risk of falls in the fully adjusted models. Increased stride length and swing time variability were the most robust predictors of falls, and the only predictors of injurious falls.
Gait, gait variability and the risk of multiple incident falls in older people: a population-based study [194] (2011)	412 participants aged between 60 and 86 years	GAITRite® system	1 year	Variability in step length and double-support phase is linearly associated with risk of multiple falls; walking speed, cadence and step-time variability are nonlinearly associated to it.
The nonlinear relationship between gait speed and falls: the maintenance of balance, independent living, intellect, and zest in the elderly of Boston study [195] (2011)	763 community-dwelling aged 78 ± 5	Time to cover 4 meters measured with a stopwatch	1,5 year	People with slow walking speed fall more indoor than other and those with fast walking speed fall more outdoor than other
Gait classification of young adults, elderly non-fallers, and elderly fallers using micro-doppler radar signals: Simulation study [205] (2017)	45 young, elderly with and without falls history	Micro-Doppler radar	/	Different walking patterns exists and could be separate by studying walking and so falls can be predicted

Study	Sample	Method of Analysis	Duration of the Follow-up	Conclusions
A prospective evaluation of balance, gait, and strength to predict falling in women with multiple sclerosis [204] (2011)	99 women with multiple sclerosis	Instrumented walkway system	1 year	Lack of stability, stand-phase asymmetries and base-of support width during gait are predictor of falls for women with MS
Increased gait variability is associated with the history of falls in patients with cerebellar ataxia [197] (2014)	48 patients with 8 types of cerebellar ataxia	6.7-meter GAITRite® walkway	6 months	Slow walking and temporal gait variability are the most relevant parameters associated to the risk of falls for patients with cerebellar ataxia
Ambulatory fall-risk assessment: Amount and quality of daily-life gait predict falls in older adults [206] (2015)	169 participants	Trunk accelerometer	6 months	The use of a daily-life accelerometer to analyze gait can help predict falls
Daily-life gait quality as predictor of falls in older people: A 1-year prospective cohort study [207] (2016)	319 participants	Trunk accelerometer	6 months to 1 year	Walking speed, stride length, stride frequency, intensity, variability, smoothness and complexity were predictive of falls.
Could local dynamic stability serve as an early predictor of falls in patients with moderate neurological gait disorders? A reliability and comparison study in healthy individuals and in patients with paresis of the lower extremities [202] (2014)	83 patients with neurological disorders (with a known risk of falls) and 40 healthy controls	Trunk accelerometer to define the Local Dynamic Stability (LDS)	/	Local Dynamic Stability can be used to differentiate fallers from non-fallers.
Local dynamic stability and variability of gait are associated with fall history in elderly subjects [203] (2012)	134 elderly	Worn accelerometer to measure LDS and gait speed	1 year	LDS and gait speed are associated and can be predictor for falling in elderly

Table 4.4. (Continued)

Study	Sample	Method of Analysis	Duration of the Follow-up	Conclusions
Relationships between walking speed, T-score and age with gait parameters in older post-menopausal women with low bone mineral density [198] (2018)	45 post-menopausal women (mean age = 67.3 years)	Motion capture cameras sampling at 100Hz	/	Gait speed explains most of the gait parameters associated with BMD which can be responsible for falls
Average in-home gait speed: investigation of a new metric for mobility and fall risk assessment of elders. [196] (2015)	16 participants residing in 14 different apartments	Kinect based gait measurement systems were installed in each apartment	11 months	Limited sample size although some participants showed significant changes over the period of monitoring largers studies need to be conducted for more conclusive evidence.
Gait variability: methods, modeling and meaning. [200] (2005)	Article review (9 studies)	Accelerometers, gyroscopes, and satellite monitoring	/	Gait variability may serve as a sensitive and clinically relevant parameter in the evaluation of mobility, fall risk and the response to therapeutic interventions.
What factors predict falls in older adults living in nursing homes: A pilot study [201] (2018)	16 adults aged 65 and over	Time to walk 40 feet (12.19-meters) measured by chronometer	6 months	Slow gait speed increased the odds of fall but is not significant

As demonstrated previously, accelerometry is another possible method of gait analysis. Patients wear sensors that use the piezoelectric effect to obtain acceleration values, which can be derived from gait parameters. For example, it was used by a study from 2015, which evaluated the association between retrospective or prospective falls and risk factors using a trunk accelerometer that 169 participants were instructed to wear for a week [206]. The portion of participants who had experienced at least one fall before baseline and those who experienced at least one fall during the study was 35.5% and 34.9% respectively. Logistic regression revealed that the quality of gait was associated with falls; thus, studying gait with a daily life accelerometer can help predict falls, as shown in Table 4.4. Moreover, the same researchers investigated the association between daily-life gait quality and fall prediction [207]. Gait characteristics were measured by a trunk accelerometer worn by 319 older participants over the course of a week. Their falls were reported during a follow-up between six months and a year. Walking speed, stride length, stride frequency, intensity, variability, smoothness, and complexity were predictive of falls.

4.5. Gait Analysis and Mortality

In light of aging demographics and increasing life expectancies at this point in history, it is vital for the clinical community to devote specialized attention and resources to care for older adults. An imperative of this care is ensuring that these individuals do not undergo unnecessary suffering and spend the remainder of their lives in a state of autonomy and dignity to the greatest extent possible. Parallel research on palliative care and the epidemiology of senescence heightens attention to the potential for gait monitoring to predict mortality in older individuals. This is vital as it helps establish a blueprint through which the goals of older adult care can be tailored and individualized to the specific needs and circumstances of each person [208].

Table 4.6 presents an overview of the relationship between gait speed and health outcomes, illustrating how variations in walking speed can serve as indicators of overall physical health and functional decline. Gait speed at the baseline of a study appears to be an effective predictor of death, as demonstrated by Rosano et al., who analyzed the increase in the risk of mortality in 3156 older adults for 8.4 years [209]. Researchers demonstrated that participants with a slow gait speed (<1.0 m/s) had higher rates of mortality than those with a gait speed greater than 1.0 m/s. A slow gait was also found to increase the risk of incident disability. The subjects were instructed to walk 15 feet (4.6 meters), and the time needed to walk this distance was recorded with a stopwatch. Researchers also wanted to determine if a lower score on the Digit Symbol Substitution Test (DSST), which is sensitive to brain damage, was associated with a higher risk of mortality. They demonstrated that individuals could exhibit a low DSST score (<27 points) without slow gait (or vice versa); however, the group with the highest risk of mortality is that in which individuals exhibited both a low DSST score and slow gait speed. A Japanese Multicenter Registry evaluated a way to predict advanced clinical outcomes for patients who had undergone transcatheter aortic valve replacement (TAVR) [210]. TAVR is a catheter used to replace a valve that is unable to open [211]. Researchers assessed the gait speed with a stopwatch while the 1256 patients walked 5 meters or 15 feet, depending on the center. There were two models of analysis used in this study. The first one categorized patients into four speed groups: normal, slow, slowest, and unable to walk. The second indicated a threshold of gait speed at 0.385 m/s. Groups from the first model exhibited a significant difference in the cumulative 1-year mortality rate, and groups from the second model showed a significant difference in survival classification. Thus, gait speed is an effective marker for predicting adverse clinical outcomes in vulnerable patients with a TAVR.

Another study investigated whether gait speed could predict mortality (and other poor outcomes, including bleeding, acute kidney injury, and stroke) for patients who had undergone a TAVR, 30 days after the operation [212]. Gait speed was assessed with a 5-meter walk, during which the time was measured with a stopwatch for 8039 participants who underwent TAVR. The mean gait speed was 0.63 m/s, which is comparatively low compared to findings from other studies, and three adapted groups were created: slow (speed < 0.5 m/s), moderate (0.5 to 0.63 m/s), and fast (greater than 0.63 m/s). Slow walkers experienced an 8.4% risk of mortality, whereas moderate and fast walkers experienced a 6.6% and 5.4% risk of mortality, respectively. After adjustment for factors including age, sex, access site, chronic lung disease, and baseline renal impairment, categorical gait speed showed significantly higher mortality at 30 days for the slowest walkers compared with normal walkers and slow walkers. Gait speed was shown to be correlated with 30-day mortality after TAVR, with slow gait speed increasing the risk of mortality.

The association between gait speed and mortality or major morbidity for patients undergoing cardiac surgery was investigated by Afilalo et al. [213]. One hundred and thirty-one participants aged 70 years and older with scheduled cardiac surgery were instructed to walk 5 meters while their gait speed was assessed using a stopwatch. Participants with a gait speed lower than 0.8 m/s were designated as slow walkers. The adjusted analysis of experiments demonstrated that slow gait speed was associated with postoperative mortality or major morbidity with an odds ratio of 3.05. Hence, slow gait speed is a good predictor of mortality after cardiac surgery (Table 4.5). A recent study on data from 50 225 walkers from 11 population-based baseline surveys in England and Scotland between 1994 and 2008 analyzed the association between all-cause mortality, cardiovascular disease, cancer mortality, and walking pace [214]. For the 49 371 that did not experience an adverse event in the first two years, the risk of all-cause and cardiovascular mortality decreased for normal- and fast-paced walkers (Table 4.5). Additionally, another study assessed the hypothesis of the association between gait speed and mortality for individuals undergoing cardiac surgery [215]. They asked 8287 patients from the Society of Thoracic Surgeons Database to walk 5 meters while being timed, establishing three groups: slow, middle, and fast. The results without adjustment are presented in Table 4.5 and demonstrate that a slow gait speed increases the risk of mortality and hospitalization. Even with adjustment, gait speed can predict mortality and rehospitalization: the hazard ratio was equal to 2.16 per 0.1 m/s decrease for mortality and equal to 1.71 per 0.1 m/s decrease for rehospitalization. Thus, regularly monitoring cardiac surgery patients can help reduce accidents (Table 4.5).

As demonstrated in the above studies, low gait speed is an effective predictor of mortality risk; however, a decline in gait speed can also predict the risk of mortality, as demonstrated by Studenski and realized with data from nine cohort studies (34 485 community-dwelling older adults) collected between 1986 and 2000 [216]. Survival was shown to decrease with decreases in gait speed, with 0.1 m/s decreases considered the threshold for significance.

One study was conducted to determine if improvement in usual gait speed in one year could be associated with better survival in older adults [217]. The study was conducted on 439 individuals aged 65 and older; six measures of health, including gait speed and global health, were tested. Gait speed was calculated as the time measured with a stopwatch to cover a 4-meter mat (Table 4.5). There were three categories to define the change in one year: improvement (0.1 m/s for the gait speed), transient improvement, and no improvement. Those with an improvement in gait speed experienced a lower risk (31.6%) of mortality eight years later than those with no improvement (49.3%); for every other health measure, there was no association with survival rate.

Table 4.5. Gait analysis and mortality

Study	Sample	Method of Analysis	Duration of the Follow-up	Conclusions
Association between lower digit symbol substitution test score and slower gait and greater risk of mortality and of developing incident disability in well-functioning older adults [209] (2008)	3156 elderly adults	Time to cover a 15-feet (4.8-meter) walk measured with a stopwatch	8.4 years	Participants with a slow gait (speed <1.0 m/s) had higher rates of mortality
Trajectories of gait speed predict mortality in well-functioning older adults: the health, aging and body composition study [208] (2013)	2364 participants (mean age = 73.5 years)	Time to cover a 20-meter walk measured with a stopwatch	8 years	A decline of 0.030 m/s per year from baseline to the last follow-up visit is associated with a 90% higher risk of mortality
Gait speed and survival in older adults [216] (2011)	34 485 community-dwelling older for 9 cohort studies	Distances calculated in meters and times in second measured by chronometer	/	Gait speed is associated with survival. A 0.1 m/s decrease is significant.
Improvement in usual gait speed predicts better survival in older adults [217] (2007)	439 adults aged 65 and older	Time to cover a 4-meter mat measured with a stopwatch	8 years	People with improvement in the gait speed in 1 year have less risk of mortality 8 years later than those with no improvement
Motoric cognitive risk syndrome and risk of mortality in older adults [218] (2016)	11 867 individuals aged over 65 years from 3 established cohort studies	Stopwatch	28 months	MCR (whose syndrome are decrease of gait speed and cognitive complaints) is associated with an increased risk of mortality
Gait speed can predict advanced clinical outcomes in patients who undergo transcatheter aortic valve replacement [210] (2017)	1256 patients	Time to cover 5-meters or 15-feet measured with a stopwatch	1 year	Gait speed is a potential marker of adverse clinical outcomes or death of patient with a transcatheter aortic valve replacement

Study	Sample	Method of Analysis	Duration of the Follow-up	Conclusions
Gait speed predicts 30-day mortality after transcatheter aortic valve replacement [212] (2016)	8039 patients that underwent transcatheter aortic valve replacement	Time to walk 5-meters measured with a stopwatch	30 days	Slow walkers (<0.5m/s) have an 8.4% risk of mortality meanwhile patients with a speed greater than the mean speed (0.63%) have a 5.4% risk
Self-rated walking pace and all-cause, cardiovascular disease and cancer mortality: individual participant pooled analysis of 50 225 walkers from 11 population British cohorts [214] (2018)	50 225 walkers	Self-rated walking speed	14 years	For the 49,371 that didn't experience an event in the first 2 years, the risk of all-cause and cardiovascular decreased for normal and fast pace.
Gait speed and mortality, hospitalization, and functional status change among hemodialysis patients: a US renal data system special study [219] (2015)	669 hemodialysis patients	Time to walk 15-feet (4.57-meters) measured with a stopwatch	Almost 2 years	A decrease in gait speed is associated with a higher risk of mortality
Gait speed and 1-year mortality following cardiac surgery: a landmark analysis from the society of thoracic surgeons adult cardiac surgery database [215] (2018)	8287 patients from the Society of Thoracic Surgeons Database (mean age: 74 years)	Time to cover 5 meters measured with a stopwatch	1 year	Slow gait speed is correlated with a higher risk of mortality and hospitalization
Gait speed as an incremental predictor of mortality and major morbidity in elderly patients undergoing cardiac surgery [213] (2010)	131 patients undergoing a cardiac surgery	Time to cover 5 meters measured with a stopwatch	/	Slow speed (<0.8 m/s) is a predictor of mortality after a cardiac surgery

Speed gait increment is not the classic scheme, but the actual final purpose of this reflection would be to determine if an intervention to improve gait would increase survival. A study with a sample of 2364 participants and a follow-up of eight years established that individuals with a gait speed decline of 0.030 m/s/year from baseline to the last follow-up visit had a 90% higher risk of mortality than those with a slower decline [209]. Gait speed was assessed with a 20-meter walk, during which participants were asked to walk at their usual pace while an interviewer was time-tracking using a stopwatch (Table 4.5). Moreover, the motoric cognitive risk (MCR) syndrome mentioned above, defined by low gait speed and cognitive impairment, is associated with increased mortality [218]. From the study, 11 867 participants aged 65 years and older, among which 836 had MCR at baseline, were followed up for 28 months. Cox and logistic regression models revealed that MCR was associated with an increased risk of mortality (Table 4.5). The association between gait speed and mortality (and other poor outcomes) for hemodialysis patients has also been investigated [219]. The usual walk speed of 669 participants was assessed with a stopwatch during a 15-foot (4.57-meter) walk (Table 4.5). Patients were classified into three groups: those who walked 0.6 m/s or faster, those who walked slower than 0.6 m/s, and those who were unable to walk 15 feet. The adjusted hazard ratios for mortality were 2.17 for patients who walked slower than 0.6 m/s and 6.93 for those who were unable to walk, compared with the participants who walked faster than 0.6 m/s. Thus, a decrease in gait speed is associated with a higher risk of mortality for patients with hemodialysis (Table 4.5).

Table 4.6. Results of the survival after one year according to the baseline speed. Data from [215]

Definition	Slow	Middle	Fast
Speed (m/s)	<0.83	0.83–1.00	>1.00
% Of Survival after 1 year	90%	95%	97%
Risk of Rehospitalization	45%	33%	27%

4.6. Gait Analysis and Cardiovascular Risk

Cardiovascular disease affects the function or structure of the heart, encompassing several disease types such as heart failure, heart valve disease, and heart attack. These diseases often arise in older individuals because of the accumulative effects of morbid conditions (e.g., diabetes, hypertension, fatty arterial plaques) that usually begin developing in young adulthood to middle age. Heart attacks, also known as myocardial infarctions, are particularly dangerous because they are often associated with general discomfort without exhibiting particularly characteristic signs or symptoms. The risk of cardiovascular disease is that, due to its often "silent" etiological path, many individuals may avoid medical attention or intervention and eventually experience preventable mortality. It is, therefore, particularly imperative to identify potential predictive links between gait monitoring and these conditions (Table 4.7).

A sample of 2725 participants (mean age = 72.7 years) in the Swedish National Study on Aging and Care in Kungsholmen was assessed to evaluate the association between cardiovascular risk factors (CRFs) such as smoking or hypertension, cardiovascular diseases (CVDs), and mobility limitations characterized by a walking speed slower than 0.8 m/s [220] (Table 4.7). Walking speed was measured by nurses with a stopwatch while participants walked 6 meters or 2.4 meters, depending on how fast they normally walked (Table 4.7). The main conclusion was that multiple CFRs and CVDs increased the risk of mobility limitations. It was shown that the increase in CVDs was highly related to an increased odds ratio of mobility limitations. The Swedish National Study on Aging and Care in Kungsholmen also realized a publication studying the association between a cardiovascular risk factor (CRF) and limitations in walking speed, chair stand, and balance [221]. They collected data on CRFs, lifestyle factors, and cognitive function for 1441 individuals free of limitations in walking speed, 1154 free of limitations in balance, and 1496 individuals free of limitations in chair stands at baseline (Table 4.7). For each individual, they calculated the walking speed by measuring the time to cover a 6-meter or 2.4-meter walk if the participants were reported to walk slowly. Limitations in walking speed were defined as walking slower than 0.8 m/s; limitations in balance were defined as being able to maintain balance for less than five seconds; and limitations in chair stands were defined as the inability to rise five times. Limitations were determined during a 3-, 6-, and 9-year follow-up. Following an analysis of the data with the Cox proportional hazards models, it was determined that the association between the Framingham general cardiovascular risk score (FRS) with walking speed limitation was evident for adults younger than 78 years old and that a higher FRS was associated with a faster decline in walking speed (Table 4.7).

Table 4.7. Gait analysis and cardiovascular risk

Study	Sample	Method of Analysis	Duration of the Follow-up	Conclusions
Association of cardiovascular burden with mobility limitation among elderly people: a population-based study [220] (2013)	2,725 participants (mean age = 72.7 years)	Measured time to cover a 6m or 2.4 m if the participants were reported to walk slowly	/	Increase of cardiovascular diseases is highly associated with increase of mobility (walking speed <0.6 m/s)
Cardiovascular risk burden and future risk of walking speed limitation in older adults [221] (2017)	1,441 individuals free of limitations in walking speed, 1154 free of limitations in balance and 1496 free of limitations in chair stands	Measured time to cover a 6 meter or 2.4 meter distance if the participants were reported to walk slowly	9 years	Framingham general cardio-vascular risk score (FRS) is associated with walking speed limitations for adults younger than 78 years old and that a higher FRS was associated with a faster decline in walking speed
Cardiovascular health is associated with physical function among older community dwelling men and women [222] (2017)	907 participants (mean age = 74)	Short Performance Physical Battery (Gait assessed by a course between 2 participants)	9 years	Walking speed is more related to cardiovascular health than balance

A recent study based on data from 907 individuals from the InCHIANTI cohort examined whether there was an association between cardiovascular health (CVH) and physical function, for which walking speed was a major measure [222]. For walking speed, the researchers concluded that it was more related to CVH than balance.

4.7. Gait Analysis and Stroke

Related to an increase in cardiovascular risk in older populations is an increase in the risk of stroke (Table 4.8). Strokes happen when a part of the brain stops functioning due to an interruption in blood flow (ischemic stroke) or the break of a blood vessel that drowns the brain cells (hemorrhagic stroke). As with cardiovascular pathologies, strokes are often "sudden onset" with little prior warning. Symptoms can range from speech, vision, and locomotion difficulties (including gait) to sudden death if risk factors and early signs are inadequately attended to. Gait monitoring can play a potentially central role in averting catastrophe if it can predict and monitor for the early development of stroke risk before it is "too late." Monitoring can also be utilized in clinical recovery if patients survive a prior stroke episode, thereby complementing existing pharmaceutical and therapeutic strategies for the clinical management of the condition.

Data from 13 048 postmenopausal women from the Women's Health Initiative was analyzed to evaluate the association between walking speed and the risk of incident ischemic stroke [223]. The gait speed was assessed by measuring the time that it took to cover a 6-meter walk at the usual speed. Researchers identified an association between slow gait speed and ischemic stroke: following adjustment, the hazard ratio was 1.69 for the slowest walking speed tertile[50] compared to the fastest. These findings are consistent with the results of a 2016 study, in which researchers analyzed the perceived walking speed of 1486 individuals without stroke history from the Sacramento Area Latino Study on Aging (SALSA) between 1998/1999 and 2010 [224]. Participants were instructed to describe their normal walking pace by choosing one of six possible responses in a form; researchers classified their responses into the categories of slow, medium, and fast. Stroke outcomes were classified into three categories: total stroke, non-fatal stroke, and fatal stroke. The results before Cox regression demonstrate that a decrease in walking speed is

---

[50] Division of study population into thirds.

associated with an increase in total stroke. In the adjusted Cox models, the hazard of total stroke was lower for medium (31%) and fast (56%) walkers than for slow walkers [224]. The conclusion was that perceived walking speed is an effective predictor for stroke risk in older Latino individuals.

Other studies related to walking speed and stroke consider the patient's ability to walk on a post-stroke basis. For example, it was investigated in a 2008 study whether studying walking speed or other gait parameters might help predict gait rehabilitation for post-stroke patients [225]. Data from 102 patients after their first-ever stroke was studied three years after the stroke. The time taken to walk a 5-meter distance was measured with a chronometer; other factors, such as the use of an assistive walking device or walking endurance, were also analyzed. The conclusion was that gait speed was significantly associated with community ambulation; however, a limitation of this finding was that this relationship was cofounded by balanced motor function, endurance, and assistive walking devices. Another study attempted to establish whether individuals with chronic stroke were able to sustain their maximum gait speed during a six-minute walk test [226]. The research was done on a sample of 48 individuals with chronic stroke. Researchers used the GAITRite® system to analyze the 6-minute and 10-meter walk tests for the participants (Table 4.8). They measured maximum gait speed, beginning and end gait speed, sustainability, the distance walk for the 6-minute walk test, and ratings of perceived exertion. The conclusion was that peak gait speed during the 6-minute walk test declined by 0.07 m/s between the beginning and the end of the test, whereas perceived exertion increased. The peak speed was slower for the 6-minute walk test than for the 10-meter walk test and faster than the beginning speed for the 6-minute walk test. However, the sustainability of the 6-minute test was the most variable for the community ambulator subgroup, indicating that the sustainability of the 6-minute and 10-meter tests must be completed for the prediction of the community ambulation potential to be correct. Another paper on 103 stroke survivors, including 67 limited walkers, compared the quality of prediction for walking speed and walking distance [227]. The tests assessed included 6-minute and 10-meter walk tests, and the conclusion was that gait speed is a more accurate predictor of walking level after a stroke than walking distance for community walking.

Table 4.8. Gait analysis and stroke

Study	Sample	Method of Analysis	Duration of the Follow-up	Conclusions
Walking speed and risk of incident ischemic stroke among postmenopausal women [223] (2008)	13,048 postmenopausal women	Measured time to cover 6 meters at usual pace	/	There is an association between slow walking speed and ischemic stroke
Perceived walking speed, measured tandem walk, incident stroke, and mortality in older Latino adults: a prospective cohort study [224] (2016)	1,486 individuals	Perceived walking speed described with a form	11-12 years	Slow walking speed increases the risk of stroke of 31% compared to medium walking speed
Community ambulation in patients with chronic stroke: how is it related to gait speed [225] (2008)	102 patients after first-ever stroke	Measured time to cover 5 meters at usual pace	/	Gait speed is significantly associated with community ambulation, but other parameters are too
Examination of sustained gait speed during extended walking in individuals with chronic stroke [226] (2013)	48 individuals with chronic stroke	GAITRite® system to analyse the 6-minute walk and the 10-meter walk	/	The sustainability of the 6-minute test was the most variable for the community ambulator subgroup meaning that the sustainability of the 6-minute and 10-meter must be completed so that the prediction of the community ambulation potential is correct
Gait velocity and walking distance to predict community walking after stroke [227] (2015)	103 stroke survivors including 67 limited walkers	Ten meters and six minutes tests with a stopwatch	/	Gait speed is a better predictor of level of walk than walking distance

4.8. Gait Analysis and Neurological Pathology

The intensifying crisis of poor mental health is a phenomenon that affects all demographic groups, but it is perhaps felt most acutely in the context of increasing loneliness among certain individuals who feel deprived of meaningful familial and social connections in light of an increasingly technological society. Older individuals are especially susceptible to loneliness and other mental health risks, considering that many are isolated from networks of kinship that are often frayed because some members of these groups have moved or passed away [228]. In addition to anxiety and depression, there is a growing burden of neuro-physiological illnesses that affect the ability of individuals, especially those in older age groups, to function at an optimal cognitive level and take full part in everyday life. It is therefore imperative to find possible connections through which gait monitoring can be used to predict illnesses and disorders of a mental or neuro-physiological nature.

Depression is a pathology also associated with gait and a decrease in walking speed. One study evaluated whether gait speed predicts depressive symptoms or vice versa [229]. Data was assessed for 1928 patients with depressive symptoms and 1855 patients with gait speed impairment from the Longitudinal Aging Study in Amsterdam. Gait speed was calculated as the time to cover a 6-meter distance with a 180° turn in the middle, measured with a stopwatch. After a 16-year follow-up, the univariate analysis revealed that gait speed at baseline could predict depressive symptoms. After adjustment for covariates, this result was only true for men. Moreover, the bidirectional associations did not share the same explanatory variables, suggesting that depression and gait speed impairment are different pathologies that can be treated in the same way.

A different study was conducted to determine if quantitative analysis of gait under single- and dual-task conditions could be used to differentiate between two neurological pathologies: progressive supranuclear palsy (PSP) and idiopathic normal-pressure hydrocephalus (iNPH) [230]. Both pathologies are known to have an impact on gait and cognitive function. Experiments were conducted on 38 patients with PSP, 27 with iNPH, and 38 with healthy controls. Gait was obtained using a pressure-sensitive carpet and measured in different situations: single task with several speeds, cognitive dual-task, and motor dual-task. Gait dysfunction and stride time variability were higher for the PSP and iNPH patients than for the healthy controls. However, stride time variability increment is more important for PSP patients than for iNPH patients. Moreover, PSP patients had worsened results when performing a cognitive dual-task and a motor dual-task. These findings suggest that more sensitive dual-task perturbation is a possible symptom of PSP, whereas increased step width and gait improvement during the motor dual-task is a possible symptom of iNPH.

Chapter 5

Discussion and Conclusion

This review has highlighted the major parameters, technologies, and correlations of gait analysis with pathologies. Many different methodologies have been analyzed in the field of gait analysis, and some are better than others as they allow more reliable detection of gait disorders. Devices that do not have body contact with individuals and those that do have been reviewed, looking at their key features and how they have been used concerning gait analysis. Finally, it has been shown how these tools can be utilized to predict the onset and development of different ailments. Gait analysis is undoubtedly a very useful tool for detecting certain ailments ahead of time. The difference between strides has been used to predict a decline in neurodegenerative diseases such as Parkinson's and Huntington's. These ailments are discoverable with a higher degree of certainty when a higher frequency of gait measures is available [196]. In recent times, this field has been demanding better diagnostic and screening technologies as older adult age groups have begun to comprise a larger portion of the global population. A lot of the current technologies available, especially the more validated ones, require a very specialized setup to capture these elements accurately. Developing an affordable system to measure these gait parameters and making it accessible enough to be used at home as well as in clinical environments would go a long way in the battle against these ailments. A system designed for this purpose should measure gait parameters such as speed, stride length, or swing time since it has been demonstrated that gait speed is independent of stride and swing time variability.

This manuscript aimed to investigate the range of pathologies that could be predicted by analyzing gait through an exploratory investigation of previous literature. As summarized in Table 5.1, the study was based on 80 publications from 1997 to 2019, of which 21 were related to decline in cognitive functions and dementia, 13 to fall prediction, ten to general predictions of adverse events, and 11 to prediction of mortality. Some of the publications evaluated the association between gait and the central nervous system, cardiovascular diseases, neurological diseases, and stroke. Seven of these papers were literary reviews, of which five focused on precise pathology.

As gait speed was the most studied parameter, 34 of the 79 publications used a stopwatch to measure the time needed to cover a defined distance. Publications that focused on other gait parameters (e.g., stance time variability, step width, stride length) mostly utilized electronic walkways with embedded sensors (e.g., GAITRite®) or accelerometers. Other methods included motion capture, insoles with embedded sensors, self-reported speed, and photo-electric cells.

Many studies involved participants older than 60 years of age or with a mean age higher than 70 years of age. Some of the papers were only analyzing healthy patients [150], but others were focused on patients with a specific pathology, such as patients who underwent surgery [145], patients with multiple sclerosis [204], patients with cerebral ataxia [197], patients that underwent a transcatheter aortic valve replacement [212], and patients with chronic stroke [226]. Finally, some studies chose to assess gait in patients with a certain disease using comparisons with healthy patients, for example, a study in which participants were either healthy or had dementia [4]. The sample size of participants varied between 16 and 50 225. The duration of the follow-up varied between 24 hours and 20 years, with many papers detailing a follow-up of one or two years. The screening test for cognitive function that is most commonly used is the Mini-Mental State Examination (MMSE), but the Montreal Cognitive Assessment (MoCA) has also been used. Cox regression was applied for many studies for the analysis of the relationship between covariates, and the results were indicated as hazard ratio {HR}, odd ratio {OR}, and risk ratio {RR}.

Gait speed is one of the most studied parameters in gait analysis. It is relatively simple to measure since only a stopwatch is needed, and it is a valid and reliable parameter when analysis is performed at the usual pace [147]. Different protocols were applied for the walking speed analysis. Some studies assessed gait speed at different rhythms: slow, usual, fast, self-selected pace, and multi-task walking (e.g., "walking while talking"). Also, some papers chose to remove the acceleration and deceleration parts of the gait trials. The length of the trials was also variable and fluctuated between 2.4 and 400 meters in different laps. In most of the studies, a cut point for gait speed was defined as a predictor of poor outcomes, but the cut point was not always consistent, and the validity and reliability of choosing particular cut points were never discussed. Hence, there is a lack of consensus concerning the walk test procedure, which complicates the interpretation of walking speed. It should also be noted that aging has an effect on gait and that it has been shown that a decline of 0.013 m/s/year is normal.

Slow gait speed (lower than 0.7 m/s) is an accurate predictor of adverse events: hospitalization, fall, need for a caregiver, and unplanned hospitalization after surgery. Slow gait speed at baseline in research was also associated with a higher risk of developing dementia and Alzheimer's diseases, poorer cognitive functions, decreased fluid cognition, poorer processing speed, short-term memory, and sustained attention. A slow gait speed could plausibly be associated with a higher risk of falls, particularly in indoor situations. Slow gait speed is also related to a higher risk of mortality and can be an accurate predictor of poor outcomes for people who underwent transcatheter aortic valve replacement (TAVR): patients who walk slower than 0.5 m/s have an 8.4% higher risk of mortality. A relationship between slow gait speed and a higher risk of cardiovascular disease has also been demonstrated. Gait speed is an excellent parameter to study stroke. First, slow gait speed increases the risk of stroke by 31%, and measuring gait speed just after a stroke can also help predict if the patient will have correct community ambulation. Finally, a slow gait speed could be a symptom of depression.

Even though there are no normative values, other studies with a follow-up of several years use the decline in gait speed as a predictor [151]. It can, for example, be a predictor of general disabilities. Moreover, the decline in gait speed is known to be related to the loss of cognitive functions and the risk of dementia. The decline of gait could appear between 7 and 12 years before the onset of cognitive functions. A decline in gait speed of 0.03 m/s/y is associated with a 90% higher risk of mortality, and there is a significantly increased risk of mortality for every 0.1 m/s decrease in gait speed.

The variability of some gait parameters, such as stance time, has also been analyzed in some studies, and it has been demonstrated to be a promising predictor for particular diseases. Stance time variability was shown to predict future disabilities; stride length variability was shown to be a predictor of poor executive function when associated with velocity; and stride length and swing time variability were shown to be associated with a higher risk of dementia. Also, gait variability appears to be closely related to falls. Individuals who fall were demonstrated to exhibit higher stride time variability frequently. Furthermore, the risk of falls was shown to increase by step length variability, stride length, and swing time variability, and it has been demonstrated that temporal gait variability is a very strong predictor of falls. Moreover, stride time variability increases for some neurological pathologies, such as progressive supranuclear palsy (PSP) and idiopathic normal-pressure hydrocephalus (iNPH).

Gait parameters can also be associated with specific functions or pathologies. For example, patients with Parkinson's disease experience reduced step length, reduced swing time, and a reduction in stability. Velocity measures, though less studied than gait speed, can sometimes be more accurate predictors of key pathologies (e.g., leg velocity in the swing phase). Also, a slow gait velocity is associated with a deficit in language and attention. Few studies have assessed gait parameters with a 400-meter walk separated into ten 40-meter laps. This is a promising area for future exploration, considering that it has been demonstrated that variation in lap time is a predictor of psychomotor and cognitive decline.

The conclusions of the reviewed literature suggest that gait could be used as a vital sign for optimized monitoring of health. The health of individuals around the world, particularly older adults, can benefit from the development and proliferation of user- and budget-friendly technologies for gait monitoring. However, work also needs to be done to better define normative values and their significant changes so that diagnoses can be reliably and validly concluded from gait analysis. At present, a rigorous gait assessment can be utilized to monitor different functions of the body but cannot yet be used to determine if a patient requires medication.

Conclusion

As technology continues to advance, gait analysis is becoming an even more powerful tool for healthcare, rehabilitation, and artificial intelligence-driven movement assessment. The integration of wearable devices, AI algorithms, and radar-based sensing is transforming the way we analyze human motion, enabling early disease detection, fall prevention, and real-time monitoring of mobility impairments.

This monograph has provided an in-depth look into the fundamentals, technological advancements, and clinical applications of gait analysis, highlighting the interdisciplinary nature of this field. The future of gait assessment lies in non-invasive, highly accurate, and intelligent monitoring systems that seamlessly integrate with healthcare solutions, making mobility assessment more accessible and effective.

Table 5.1. Summary of the methods used and the pathologies assessed

Type of pathology	Stopwatch	Electronics with embedded sensors	Motion capture systems	Force insoles	Accelerometers	Self-reported gait parameters	Literary review	Photoelectric cells	Radar	Other	Total
General predictions	[150, 144, 146, 151, 145]	/	[13]	/	/	/	[147, 148]	[152]	/	/	10
Decline in cognitive function and dementia	[156, 162, 170, 171, 172, 166, 157, 161, 168, 167]	[4, 165, 169, 174, 160]	/	/	/	[149]	[163, 159, 158, 173]	[155]	[81]	/	21
Association with CNS	[188]	[187, 179, 180, 183, 184, 185]	/	/	/	/	[181]	/	/	[186, 189, 190, 192, 178, 182, 193]	15
Falls prediction	[195, 201] (chronometer)	[199, 194, 204, 197]	[198]	[20]	[206, 207, 202, 203]	/	/	/	[205]	/	13
Mortality	[209, 208, 216, 217, 218, 212, 214, 215, 213, 211]	/	/	/	/	[219]	/	/	/	/	11
Cardio-vascular disease	[221, 222, 223]	/	/	/	/	/	/	/	/	/	3
Stroke	[224, 226, 229]	[227]	/	/	/	[225]	/	/	/	/	5
Neurological disease	[230]	[56]	/	/	/	/	/	/	/	/	2
Total	34	17	2	1	4	3	7	2	2	7	80

Looking ahead, researchers and engineers must address key challenges such as data privacy, sensor accuracy, and real-world implementation of AI-driven gait monitoring. By fostering collaboration between engineers, medical professionals, and AI specialists, the future of gait analysis will continue to evolve, improving health outcomes, mobility independence, and quality of life for individuals worldwide.

This monograph serves as a foundation for future exploration, encouraging further research, innovation, and the development of next-generation gait analysis tools that will shape the future of healthcare and human movement science.

References

[1] Kharb, A., V. Saini, Y. K. Jain and S. Dhiman, "A Review of Gait Cycle and its Parameters," *International Journal of Computational Engineering and Management,* vol. 13, p. 78–83, 2011.

[2] Bridenbaugh, S. A. and R. W. Kressig, "Laboratory Review: The Role of Gait Analysis in Seniors' Mobility and Fall Prevention," *Gerontology,* vol. 57, no. 3, p. 256–264, 2011.

[3] Lord, S., B. Galna, S. Coleman, A. Yarnall, D. Burn and L. Rochester, "Cognition and Gait Show a Selective Pattern of Association Dominated by Phenotype in Incident Parkinson's Disease," *Frontiers in Aging Neuroscience,* vol. 6, p. 249, 2014.

[4] Verghese, J., C. Wang, R. B. Lipton, R. Holtzer and X. Xue, "Quantitative Gait Dysfunction and Risk of Cognitive Decline and Dementia," *Journal of Neurology, Neurosurgery and Psychiatry,* vol. 78, no. 9, p. 929–935, 2007.

[5] Chen, M. A., "Frailty and Cardiovascular Disease: Potential Role of Gait Speed in Surgical Risk Stratification in Older Adults," *Journal of Geriatric Cardiology,* vol. 12, no. 1, p. 44–56, 2015.

[6] Tao, W., T. Liu, R. Zheng and H. Feng, "Gait Analysis Using Wearable Sensors," *Sensors,* vol. 12, no. 2, p. 2255–2283, 2012.

[7] Jarchi, D., J. Pope, T. Lee, L. Tamjidi, A. Mirzaei and S. Sanei, "A Review on Accelerometry-based Gait Analysis and Emerging Clinical Applications," *IEEE Reviews in Biomedical Engineering,* vol. 11, p. 177–194, 2018.

[8] "Phases of the Normal Gait Cycle," [Online]. Available: https://www.researchgate.net/figure/Phases-of-the-normal-gait-cycle_fig3_309362425. [Accessed 21 November 2023].

[9] Helbostad, J. and R. Moe-Nilssen, "The Effect of Gait Speed on Lateral Balance Control during Walking in Healthy Elderly," *Gait and Posture,* vol. 18, p. 27–36, 2003.

[10] Schimpl, M. et al., "Association between Walking Speed and Age in Healthy, Free-Living Individuals Using Mobile Accelerometry—A Cross-Sectional Study," *Plos One,* vol. 6, no. 8, p. e23299, 2011.

[11] "Portable Gait Analysis System | GAITRite," [Online]. Available: https://www.gaitrite.com/. [Accessed 22 March 2022].

[12] Okinaka, H. et al., "Gait Classification of Healthy Young and Elderly Adults Using Micro-Doppler Radar Remote Sensing," in *2018 Joint 10th International Conference on Soft Computing and Intelligent Systems (SCIS),* Toyama, 2018.

[13] Jerome, G. J., S. Ko, D. Kauffman, S. A. Studenski, L. Ferrucci and E. M. Simonsick, "Gait Characteristics Associated with Walking Speed Decline in Older Adults: Results from the Baltimore Longitudinal Study of Aging," *Archives of Gerontology and Geriatrics,* vol. 60, no. 2, p. 239–243, 2015.

[14] Viccaro, L. J., S. Perera and S. A. Studenski, "Is Timed Up and Go Better Than Gait Speed in Predicting Health, Function, and Falls in Older Adults?," *Journal of the American Geriatrics Society,* vol. 59, no. 5, p. 887–892, 2011.

[15] Brach, J. S., S. Perera, S. Studenski, M. Katz, C. Hall and J. Verghese, "Meaningful Change in Measures of Gait Variability in Older Adults," *Gait and Posture,* vol. 31, no. 2, p. 175–179, 2010.

[16] Rennie, L., N. Löfgren, R. Moe-Nilssen, A. Opheim, E. Dietrichs and E. Franzén, "The Reliability of Gait Variability Measures for Individuals with Parkinson's Disease and Healthy Older Adults – The Effect of Gait Speed," *Gait and Posture,* vol. 62, p. 505–509, 2018.

[17] Beauchet, O. et al., "Guidelines for Assessment of Gait and Reference Values for Spatiotemporal Gait Parameters in Older Adults: The Biomathics and Canadian Gait Consortiums Initiative," *Frontiers in Human Neuroscience,* vol. 11, p. 353, 2017.

[18] Kubicki, A., "Functional Assessment in Older Adults: Should we use Timed Up and Go or Gait Speed Test?," *Neuroscience Letters,* vol. 577, p. 89–94, 2014.

[19] Brach, J. S., S. A. Studenski, S. Perera, J. M. van Swearingen and A. B. Newman, "Gait Variability and the Risk of Incident Mobility Disability in Community-Dwelling Older Adults," *The Journals of Gerontology Series A: Biological Sciences and Medical Sciences,* vol. 62, no. 9, p. 983–988, 2007.

[20] Hausdorff, J. M., D. A. Rios and H. K. Edelberg, "Gait Variability and Fall Risk in Community-living Older Adults: A 1-year Prospective Study," *Archives of Physical Medicine and Rehabilitation,* vol. 82, no. 8, p. 1050–1056, 2001.

[21] Autenrieth, C. S. et al., "Decline in Gait Performance Detected by an Electronic Walkway System in 907 Older Adults of the Population-Based KORA-Age Study," *Gerontology,* vol. 59, no. 2, p. 165–173, 2013.

[22] McDonough, A. L., M. Batavia, F. C. Chen, S. Kwon and J. Ziai, "The Validity and Reliability of the GAITRite System's Measurements: A Preliminary Evaluation," *Archives of Physical Medicine and Rehabilitation,* vol. 82, no. 3, p. 419–425, 2001.

[23] "Stepscan," Stepscan Technologies INC, [Online]. Available: https://stepscan.com/. [Accessed 2022].

[24] Walford, A. et al., "Development of a Gait Assessment Protocol for Elderly Veterans with Cognitive Decline, Using an Instrumented Walkway," *Journal of Military, Veteran and Family Health,* vol. 5, no. 1, p. 49–57, 2019.

[25] "The Zeno Walkway Gait Analysis System," [Online]. Available: https://www.protokinetics.com/zeno-walkway/. [Accessed 22 March 2022].

[26] Vallabhajosula, S., S. K. Humphrey, A. J. Cook and J. E. Freund, "Concurrent Validity of the Zeno Walkway for Measuring Spatiotemporal Gait Parameters in Older Adults," *Journal of Geriatric Physical Therapy,* vol. 42, no. 3, p. E42–E50, 2019.

References

[27] "OptoGait | Microgate," [Online]. Available: https://medical.microgate.it/en/products/optogait. [Accessed 21 December 2023].

[28] "The System on Treadmill | Microgate," Microgate, [Online]. Available: https://medical.microgate.it/en/products/optogait/system-treadmill. [Accessed 2022].

[29] Item-Glatthorn, J. F. and N. A. Maffiuletti, "Clinical Assessment of Spatiotemporal Gait Parameters in Patients and Older Adults," *Journal of Visualized Experiments,* vol. 93, p. e51878, 2014.

[30] Lienhard, K., D. Schneider and N. A. Maffiuletti, "Validity of the Optogait Photoelectric System for the Assessment of Spatiotemporal Gait Parameters," *Medical Engineering and Physics,* vol. 35, p. 500–504, 2013.

[31] "Dynamic Gait Analysis on the Treadmill," Zebris Medical GmbH, [Online]. Available: https://www.zebris.de/en/medical/dynamic-gait-analysis-on-the-treadmill. [Accessed 22 March 2022].

[32] "Rehawalk® Pressure Treadmill for Treatment of Gait Disorders - Noraxon USA," 2022. [Online]. Available: https://www.noraxon.com/our-products/rehawalk-pressure-treadmill/. [Accessed 7 February 2024].

[33] Van Alsenoy, K., A. Thomson and A. Burnett, "Reliability and Validity of the Zebris FDM-THQ Instrumented Treadmill During Running Trials," *Sports Biomechanics,* vol. 18, no. 5, pp. 501-514, 2018.

[34] Higginson, B. K., "Methods of Running Gait Analysis," *Current Sports Medicine Reports,* vol. 8, no. 3, p. 136–141, 2009.

[35] "Life Sciences | Vicon Motion Capture for Biomechanics," [Online]. Available: https://www.vicon.com/applications/life-sciences/. [Accessed 21 December 2023].

[36] Lee, I. and S. Park, "A Comparison of Gait Characteristics in the Elderly People, People with Knee Pain, and People who are Walker Dependent People," *Journal of Physical Therapy Science,* vol. 25, no. 8, p. 973–976, 2013.

[37] Kobayashi, Y., H. Hobara, T. A. Heldoorn, M. Kouchi and M. Mochimaru, "Age-independent and Age-dependent Sex Differences in Gait Pattern Determined by Principal Component Analysis," *Gait and Posture,* vol. 46, pp. 11-17, 2016.

[38] Windows Central, [Online]. Available: https://www.ebay.ca/itm/143546365751. [Accessed 14 October 2024].

[39] Eltoukhy, M., J. Oh, C. Kuenze and J. Signorile, "Improved Kinect-based Spatiotemporal and Kinematic Treadmill Gait Assessment," *Gait and Posture,* vol. 51, p. 77–83, 2017.

[40] Tychola, K., I. Tsimperidis and G. Papakostas, "On 3D Reconstruction Using RGB-D Cameras," *Digital,* vol. 2, no. 3, p. 401–421, 2022.

[41] Fosty, B. et al., "Accuracy and Reliability of the RGB-D Camera for Measuring Walking Speed on a Treadmill," *Gait and Posture,* vol. 48, p. 113–119, 2016.

[42] "Biomechanics and Life Sciences | Kistler," Kistler, [Online]. Available: https://www.kistler.com/INT/en/biomechanics-and-life-sciences/C00000187. [Accessed 21 December 2023].

[43] Faber, G. S. et al., "A Force Plate Based Method for the Calibration of Force/Torque Sensors," *Journal of Biomechanics,* vol. 45, no. 7, p. 1332–1338, 2012.

[44] "Multi-Axis Force Plates | AMTI," [Online]. Available: https://www.amti.biz/product-line/force-plates/. [Accessed 21 December 2023].
[45] Verniba, D., M. E. Vergara and W. H. Gage, "Force Plate Targeting has No Effect on Spatiotemporal Gait Measures and their Variability in Young and Healthy Population," *Gait and Posture,* vol. 41, no. 2, p. 551–556, 2015.
[46] Morita, P. et al., "Comparative Analysis of Gait Speed Estimation Using Wideband and Narrowband Radars, Thermal Camera, and Motion Tracking Suit Technologies," *Journal of Healthcare Informatics Research,* vol. 4, no. 3, p. 215–237, 2020.
[47] Lu, X. and A. Memari, "Application of Infrared Thermography for In-situ Determination of Building Envelope Thermal Properties," *Journal of Building Engineering,* vol. 26, p. 100885, 2019.
[48] Slemenšek, J. et al., "Human Gait Activity Recognition Machine Learning Methods," *Sensors,* vol. 23, no. 2, p. 745, 2023.
[49] "Center for Biometrics and Security Research," [Online]. Available: http://www.cbsr.ia.ac.cn/english/Gait%20Databases.asp. [Accessed 12 April 2022].
[50] Jiang, X., Y. Zhang, Q. Yang, B. Deng and H. Wang, "Millimeter-Wave Array Radar-Based Human Gait Recognition Using Multi-Channel Three-Dimensional Convolutional Neural Network," *Sensors,* vol. 20, no. 19, p. 5466, 2020.
[51] Hornsteiner, C. and J. Detlefsen, "Extraction of Features Related to Human Gait Using a Continuous-Wave Radar," in *German Microwave Conference*, 2008.
[52] Yang, L., G. Chen and G. Li, "Classification of Personnel Targets with Baggage using Dual-band Radar," *Remote Sensing,* vol. 9, no. 6, p. 594, 2017.
[53] Otero, M., "Application of a Continuous Wave Radar for Human Gait Recognition," in *Proceedings Volume 5809 - Signal Processing, Sensor Fusion, and Target Recognition XIV*, Orlando, 2005.
[54] Anderson, M. and R. Rogers, "Micro-Doppler analysis of Multiple Frequency Continuous Wave Radar Signatures," in *Proceedings Volume 6547 Radar Sensor Technology XI*, Orlando, 2007.
[55] Zhang, J., "Basic Gait Analysis Based on Continuous Wave Radar," *Gait and Posture,* vol. 36, no. 4, p. 667–671, 2012.
[56] Qiu, Z., D. Li and W. Jiang, "Study of Continuous Wave Radar for Human Motion Characteristics Measurement," in *IEEE 10th International Conference on Signal Processing Proceedings*, 2010.
[57] Ma, X., R. Zhao, X. Liu, H. Kuang and M. A. A. Al-qaness, "Classification of Human Motions Using Micro-Doppler Radar in the Environments with Micro-Motion Interference," *Sensors,* vol. 19, no. 11, p. 2598, 2019.
[58] Saho, K. et al., "Estimation of Gait Parameters from Trunk Movement Measured by Doppler Radar," *IEEE Journal of Electromagnetics, RF and Microwaves in Medicine and Biology,* vol. 6, no. 4, p. 461–469, 2022.
[59] Shi, Y. et al., "Robust Gait Recognition Based on Deep CNNs With Camera and Radar Sensor Fusion," *IEEE Internet of Things Journal,* vol. 10, no. 12, p. 10817–10832, 2023.

References

[60] Geisheimer, J. L., W. S. Marshall and E. Greneker, "A Continuous-Wave (CW) Radar for Gait Analysis," *Conference Record of Thirty-Fifth Asilomar Conference on Signals, Systems and Computers,* vol. 1, p. 834–838, 2001.

[61] Boroomand, A., G. Shaker, P. P. Morita, A. Wong and J. Boger, "Autonomous Gait Speed Estimation using 24GHz FMCW Radar Technology," in *2018 IEEE EMBS International Conference on Biomedical and Health Informatics,* 2018.

[62] van Dorp, P. and F. C. A. Groen, "Human Walking Estimation with Radar," *IEEE Proceedings - Radar, Sonar and Navigation,* vol. 150, no. 5, p. 356, 2003.

[63] Hsu, C.-Y., Y. Liu, Z. Kabelac, R. Hristov, D. Katabi and C. Liu, "Extracting Gait Velocity and Stride Length from Surrounding Radio Signals," in *Proceedings of the 2017 CHI Conference on Human Factors in Computing Systems,* 2017.

[64] Abedi, H., A. Ansariyan, P. P. Morita, A. Wong, J. Boger and G. Shaker, "AI-powered Non-contact In-home Gait Monitoring and Activity Recognition System Based on mm-wave FMCW Radar and Cloud Computing," *IEEE Internet of Things Journal,* 2023.

[65] Abedi, H., A. Ansariyan, P. Morita, A. Wong, J. Boger and G. Shaker, "In-home Activity Monitoring Using Radars," *Journal of Computational Vision and Imaging Systems,* vol. 8, no. 1, p. 5–6, 2022.

[66] Abedi, H., J. Boger, P. Morita, A. Wong and G. Shaker, "Hallway Gait Monitoring Using Novel Radar Signal Processing and Unsupervised Learning," *Sensors,* vol. 22, no. 15, pp. 15133-15145, 2022.

[67] Wang, D., J. Park, H.-J. Kim, K. Lee and C. S. H., "Noncontact Extraction of Biomechanical Parameters in Gait Analysis Using a Multi-Input and Multi-Output Radar Sensor," *IEEE Access,* pp. 1-1, 2021.

[68] Niazi, U., S. Hazra, A. Santra and R. Weigel, "Radar-Based Efficient Gait Classification using Gaussian Prototypical Networks," in *2021 IEEE Radar Conference,* Atlanta, 2021.

[69] Abedi, H., J. Boger, P. P. Morita, A. Wong and G. Shaker, "Hallway Gait Monitoring System Using an In-package Integrated Dielectric Lens Paired with a mm-wave Radar," *Sensors,* vol. 23, no. 1, p. 71, 2022.

[70] Abedi, H., P. P. Morita, J. Boger, A. Wong and G. Shaker, "In-package Integrated Dielectric Lens Paired with a MIMO mm-wave Radar for Corridor Gait Monitoring," in *2021 IEEE International Symposium on Antennas and Propagation and USNC-URSI Radio Science Meeting,* 2021.

[71] di Renzo, M., R. M. Buehrer and J. Torres, "Pulse Shape Distortion and Ranging Accuracy in UWB-Based Body Area Networks for Full-Body Motion Capture and Gait Analysis," in *IEEE Globecom 2007-2007 IEEE Global Telecommunications Conference,* 2007.

[72] Choi, J. W., X. Quan and S. H. Cho, "Bi-Directional Passing People Counting System Based on IR-UWB Radar Sensors," *IEEE Internet of Things Journal,* vol. 5, no. 2, p. 512–522, 2018.

[73] Saho, K., S. T., T. Sato, K. Inoue and T. Fukuda, "Pedestrian Imaging Using UWB Doppler Radar Interferometry," *IEICE Transactions on Communications,* Vols. E96-B, no. 2, p. 613–623, 2013.

[74] Rana, S. P., M. Dey, M. Ghavami and S. Dudley, "Non-Contact Human Gait Identification Through IR-UWB Edge-Based Monitoring Sensor," *IEEE Sensors Journal,* vol. 19, no. 20, p. 9282–9293, 2019.

[75] Lau, B., S. Haider, A. Boroomand, G. Shaker, J. Boger and P. Morita, "Gait Speed Tracking System Using UWB Radar," in *12th European Conference on Antennas and Propagation,* London, 2018.

[76] Wang, Y. and A. E. Fathy, "Range-time-frequency Representation of a Pulse Doppler Radar Imaging System for Indoor Localization and Classification," in *IEEE Topical Conference on Wireless Sensors and Sensor Networks,* 2013.

[77] Wang, F., M. Skubic, M. Rantz and P. Cuddihy, "Quantitative Gait Measurement With Pulse-Doppler Radar for Passive In-Home Gait Assessment," *IEEE Transactions on Biomedical Engineering,* vol. 61, no. 9, p. 2434–2443, 2014.

[78] Yardibi, T. et al., "Gait Characterization via Pulse-Doppler Radar," in *IEEE International Conference on Pervasive Computing and Communications Workshops (PERCOM Workshops),* 2011.

[79] Phillips, C. E. et al., "Radar Walk Detection in the Apartments of Elderly," in *2012 Annual International Conference of the IEEE Engineering in Medicine and Biology Society,* 2012.

[80] Alshamaa, D., A. Chkeir, R. Soubra and B. Dauriac, "A Smart Radar System for Automatic Functional Capacity Tests," in *2019 3rd International Conference on Bio-Engineering for Smart Technologies,* 2019.

[81] Alshamaa, D., R. Soubra and A. Chkeir, "A Radar Sensor for Automatic Gait Speed Analysis in Walking Tests," *Sensors,* vol. 21, no. 12, pp. 13886-13894, 2021.

[82] Shah, S. et al., "Sensor Fusion for Identification of Freezing of Gait Episodes Using Wi-Fi and Radar Imaging," *IEEE Sensors Journal,* vol. 20, no. 23, p. 14410–14422, 2020.

[83] Abedi, H., G. Shaker, J. Boger, P. Morita and A. Wong, "Use of High-Frequency Radar for Gait Monitoring," *American Journal of Biomedical Science and Research,* vol. 6, no. 2, 2019.

[84] Abedi, H., P. P. Morita, J. Boger, A. Wong and G. Shaker, "Unsupervised Learning for Hallway Gait Analysis using FMCW Radar," in *2022 IEEE International Symposium on Antennas and Propagation and USNC-URSI Radio Science Meeting,* 2022.

[85] Abedi, H., A. Ansariyan, P. P. Morita, J. Boger, A. Wong and G. Shaker, "Sequential Deep Learning for In-home Activity Monitoring Using mm-wave FMCW Radar," in *2021 IEEE International Symposium on Antennas and Propagation and USNC-URSI Radio Science Meeting,* 2021.

[86] Abedi, H. et al., "On the Use of an In-Package Dielectric Lens Antenna for Radar-based Applications," *IEEE Transactions on Components, Packaging and Manufacturing Technology,* 2024.

[87] Vienne, A., R. P. Barrois, S. Buffat, D. Ricard and P. P. Vidal, "Inertial Sensors to Assess Gait Quality in Patients with Neurological Disorders: A Systematic Review of Technical and Analytical Challenges," *Frontiers in Psychology,* vol. 8, p. 817, 2017.

References

[88] Subramaniam, S., A. Faisal and M. Deen, "Wearable Sensor Systems for Fall Risk Assessment: A Review," *Front Digit Health,* vol. 4, p. 921506, 14 July 2022.

[89] "G-WALK | Wearable Inertial Sensor for Motion Analysis | BTS," [Online]. Available: https://www.btsbioengineering.com/products/g-walk/. [Accessed 21 November 2023].

[90] Ridder, R., J. Lebleu, T. Willems, C. Blaiser, C. Detrembleur and R. P., "Concurrent Validity of a Commercial Wireless Trunk Triaxial Accelerometer System for Gait Analysis," *Journal of Sport Rehabilitation,* vol. 28, no. 6, 2019.

[91] Pau, M., B. Leban, G. Collu and G. M. Migliaccio, "Effect of Light and Vigorous Physical Activity on Balance and Gait of Older Adults," *Archives of Gerontology and Geriatrics,* vol. 59, no. 3, p. 568–573, 2014.

[92] "Physilog | Inertial Measurement Unit (IMU)," MindMaze Group SA, [Online]. Available: https://research.gaitup.com/physilog/. [Accessed 22 March 2022].

[93] Molengraft, J., S. Nimmala, B. Mariani, K. Aminian, C. Büla and P. J., "Wireless 6D Inertial Measurement Platform for Ambulatory Gait Monitoring," in *Proceedings of the 6th international workshop on Wearable, Micro and Nanosystems for Personalised Health,* 2009.

[94] Mariani, B., C. Hoskovec, S. Rochat, C. Büla, J. Penders and K. Aminian, "3D Gait Assessment in Young and Elderly Subjects using Foot-worn Inertial Sensors," *Journal of Biomechanics,* vol. 43, no. 15, p. 2999–3006, 2010.

[95] Perera, S., S. H. Mody, R. C. Woodman and S. A. Studenski, "Meaningful Change and Responsiveness in Common Physical Performance Measures in Older Adults," *Journal of the American Geriatrics Society,* vol. 54, no. 5, p. 743–749, 2006.

[96] Mariani, B., H. Rouhani, X. Crevoisier and K. Aminian, "Quantitative Estimation of Foot-flat and Stance Phase of Gait using Foot-worn Inertial Sensors," *Gait and Posture,* vol. 37, no. 2, p. 229–234, 2013.

[97] Ganea, R. et al., "Gait Assessment in Children with Duchenne Muscular Dystrophy During Long-distance Walking," *Journal of Child Neurology,* vol. 27, no. 1, p. 30–38, 2012.

[98] Brégou Bourgeois, A., B. Mariani, K. Aminian, P. Y. Zambelli and C. J. Newman, "Spatio-temporal Gait Analysis in Children with Cerebral Palsy using Foot-worn Inertial Sensors," *Gait and Posture,* vol. 39, no. 1, p. 436–442, 2014.

[99] "Wearable Sensors - APDM Wearable Technologies," APDM Wearable Technologies, [Online]. Available: https://apdm.com/mobility/. [Accessed 1 June 2022].

[100] Mancini, M., L. King, A. Salarian, L. Holmstrom, J. McNames and F. B. Horak, "Mobility Lab to Assess Balance and Gait with Synchronized Body-worn Sensors," *Journal of Bioengineering and Biomedical Science,* vol. 1, p. 007, 2011.

[101] Morris, R., S. Stuart, G. Mcbarron, P. C. Fino, M. Mancini and C. Curtze, "Validity of Mobility Lab for Gait Assessment in Young Adults, Older Adults and Parkinson's Disease," *Physiological Measurement,* vol. 40, no. 9, p. 095003, 2019.

[102] Washabaugh, E. P., T. Kalyanaraman, P. G. Adamczyk, E. S. Claflin and C. Krishnan, "Validity and Repeatability of Inertial Measurement Units for Measuring Gait Parameters," *Gait and Posture,* vol. 55, p. 87–93, 2017.

[103] Morris, R. et al., "Cognitive Associations with Comprehensive Gait and Static Balance Measures in Parkinson's Disease," *Parkinsonism and Related Disorders,* vol. 69, p. 104–110, 2019.

[104] Soczawa-Stronczyk, A. A., M. Bocian, H. Wdowicka and J. Malin, "Topological Assessment of Gait Synchronisation in Overground Walking Groups," *Human Movement Science,* vol. 66, p. 541–553, 2019.

[105] Riva, F., M. C. Bisi and R. Stagni, "Gait Variability and Stability Measures: Minimum Number of Strides and Within-session Reliability," *Computers in Biology and Medicine,* vol. 50, p. 9–13, 2014.

[106] Hollman, J. H., M. K. Watkins, A. C. Imhoff, C. E. Braun, K. A. Akervik and D. K. Ness, "A Comparison of Variability in Spatiotemporal Gait Parameters between Treadmill and Overground Walking Conditions," *Gait and Posture,* vol. 43, p. 204–209, 2016.

[107] "Letsense Group - Free4Act Technology," [Online]. Available: http://www.letsense.net/free4act_eng.php. [Accessed 29 November 2023].

[108] Benedetti, M. G. et al., "Gait Measures in Patients With and Without AFO for Equinus Varus/Drop Foot," in *IEEE International Symposium on Medical Measurements and Applications, Proceedings,* 2011.

[109] "Axivity | Product," [Online]. Available: https://axivity.com/product/ax3. [Accessed 29 November 2023].

[110] Godfrey, A., S. Del Din, G. Barry, J. C. Mathers and L. Rochester, "Instrumenting Gait with an Accelerometer: A System and Algorithm Examination," *Medical Engineering and Physics,* vol. 37, no. 4, p. 400–407, 2015.

[111] Del Din, S., A. Godfrey and L. Rochester, "Validation of an Accelerometer to Quantify a Comprehensive Battery of Gait Characteristics in Healthy Older Adults and Parkinson's Disease: Toward Clinical and at Home Use," *IEEE Journal of Biomedical and Health Informatics,* vol. 20, no. 3, p. 838–847, 2016.

[112] Del Din, S. et al., "Measuring Gait with an Accelerometer-based Wearable: Influence of Device Location, Testing Protocol and Age," *Physiological Measurement,* vol. 37, no. 10, p. 1785, 2016.

[113] "MoveMonitor | Ambulatory Monitoring of Physical Activity for up to 14 Days," [Online]. Available: https://www.mcroberts.nl/products/movemonitor/. [Accessed 22 March 2022].

[114] Houdijk, H., F. M. Appelman, J. M. van Velzen, L. H. v. van der Woude and C. A. M. van Bennekom, "Validity of DynaPort GaitMonitor for Assessment of Spatiotemporal Parameters in Amputee Gait," *The Journal of Rehabilitation Research and Development,* vol. 45, no. 9, p. 1335, 2008.

[115] De Groot, M. H. et al., "A Flexed Posture in Elderly Patients is Associated with Impairments in Postural Control During Walking," *Gait and Posture,* vol. 39, no. 2, p. 767–772, 2014.

[116] "Wearable Sensor Technology," [Online]. Available: https://shimmersensing.com/. [Accessed 22 March 2022].

[117] Avvenuti, M. et al., "Smart Shoe-Assisted Evaluation of Using a Single Trunk/Pocket-Worn Accelerometer to Detect Gait Phases," *Sensors,* vol. 18, no. 11, p. 3811, 2018.

[118] Greene, B. R., T. G. Foran, D. McGrath, E. P. Doheny, A. Burns and B. Caulfield, "A Comparison of Algorithms for Body-Worn Sensor-Based Spatiotemporal Gait Parameters to the GAITRite Electronic Walkway," *Journal of Applied Biomechanics,* vol. 28, no. 3, p. 349–355, 2012.

[119] "Inertial Measurement Unit | Technaid - Leading Motion," [Online]. Available: https://www.technaid.com/products/inertial-measurement-unit-tech-imu-biomechanichs/. [Accessed 2023 November 29].

[120] Scaglioni-Solano, P. and L. F. Aragón-Vargas, "Age-related Differences when Walking Downhill on Different Sloped Terrains," *Gait and Posture,* vol. 41, no. 1, p. 153–158, 2015.

[121] Scaglioni-Solano, P. and L. F. Aragón-Vargas, "Gait Characteristics and Sensory Abilities of Older Adults are Modulated by Gender," *Gait and Posture,* vol. 42, no. 1, pp. 54-59, 2015.

[122] Guimaraes, R. and B. Isaacs, "Characteristics of the Gait in Old People who Fall," *International Rehabilitation Medicine,* vol. 2, no. 4, p. 177–180, 1980.

[123] "Microstone Co., Ltd. - Opening up the Future with Motion Sensors and Vibration Sensors," [Online]. Available: https://www.microstone.co.jp/. [Accessed 29 November 2023].

[124] Wang, H. et al., "Reliability of Lower Leg Proximal End and Forefoot Kinematics During Different Paces of Barefoot Racewalking on a Treadmill Using a Motion Recorder (MVP-RF8-BC)," *The Journal of Physical Therapy Science,* vol. 28, no. 4, p. 1155–1157, 2016.

[125] Misu, S. et al., "Association between Toe Flexor Strength and Spatiotemporal Gait Parameters in Community-dwelling Older People," *Journal of NeuroEngineering and Rehabiliation,* vol. 11, no. 1, p. 1–7, 2014.

[126] Aminian, K., B. Najafi, C. Büla, P. F. Leyvraz and P. Robert, "Spatio-temporal Parameters of Gait Measured by an Ambulatory System Using Miniature Gyroscopes," *Journal of Biomechanics,* vol. 35, no. 5, p. 689–699, 2002.

[127] Wong, W., M. Wong and K. Lo, "Clinical Applications of Sensors for Human Posture and Movement Analysis: A Review," *Prosthetics and Orthotics International,* vol. 31, no. 1, pp. 62-75, 2007.

[128] Sabatini, A. M., C. Martelloni, S. Scapellato and F. Cavallo, "Assessment of Walking Features from Foot Inertial Sensing," *IEEE Transactions on Biomedical Engineering,* vol. 52, no. 3, p. 486–494, 2005.

[129] "Intelligent Device for Energy Expenditure and Activity," MiniSun, [Online]. Available: http://www.minisun.com/ideea.htm. [Accessed 22 March 2022].

[130] Rigsby, M., "Validation of the MiniSun IDEEA Data Recorder for the Analysis of Walking on Uneven Ground," *Graduate Theses and Dissertations,* p. 489, 2011.

[131] "Footmoov – The Footwear Revolution," [Online]. Available: https://www.footmoov.com/. [Accessed 21 December 2023].

[132] Hacker, S., C. Kalkbrenner, M.-E. Algorri and R. Blechschmidt-Trapp, "Gait Analysis with IMU Gaining New Orientation Information of the Lower Leg," in *International Conference of Biomedical Electronics and Devices,* 2014.

[133] Bamberg, S. J. M., A. Y. Benbasat, D. M. Scarborough, D. E. Krebs and J. A. Paradiso, "Gait Analysis using a Shoe-integrated Wireless Sensor System," *IEEE*

Transactions on Information Technology in Biomedicine, vol. 12, no. 4, p. 413–423, 2008.

[134] "Homepage - FeetMe," [Online]. Available: https://feetmehealth.com/. [Accessed 21 December 2023].

[135] Farid, L. et al., "FeetMe® Monitor-connected Insoles are a Valid and Reliable Alternative for the Evaluation of Gait Speed after Stroke," *Topics in Stroke Rehabilitation,* vol. 28, no. 2, p. 127–134, 2021.

[136] "RunScribe - Wearable IMU - Gait Analysis," [Online]. Available: https://runscribe.com/red/. [Accessed 8 February 2024].

[137] García-Pinillos, F., J. M. Chicano-Gutiérrez, E. J. Ruiz-Malagón and L. E. Roche-Seruendo, "Influence of RunScribeTM Placement on the Accuracy of Spatiotemporal Gait Characteristics During Running," *Journal of Sports Engineering and Technology,* vol. 234, no. 1, p. 11–18, 2020.

[138] "Sensor Insoles for Clinical Grade Mobile Gait and Motion Analysis," [Online]. Available: https://moticon.com/. [Accessed 21 December 2023].

[139] Braun, B. J. et al., "Validation and Reliability Testing of a New, Fully Integrated Gait Analysis Insole," *Journal of Foot and Ankle Research,* vol. 8, no. 1, p. 1–7, 2015.

[140] "The Zebris FDM-S Multifunction Force Measuring Plate [Exhibition catalogue]," Zebris Medical GmbH, Isny im Allgäu, 2007.

[141] "Xprecia Stride," Universal Biosensors, 2024. [Online]. Available: https://universalbiosensors.com/products/xprecia-stride/. [Accessed 9 October 2024].

[142] Beckwée, D. et al., "Validity and Test-Retest Reliability of the Stride Analyzer in People with Knee Osteoarthritis," *Gait and Posture,* vol. 49, p. 155–158, 2016.

[143] Government of Canada, "Aging and Chronic Diseases: A Profile of Canadian Seniors," [Online]. Available: https://www.canada.ca/en/public-health/services/publications/diseases-conditions/aging-chronic-diseases-profile-canadian-seniors-report.html. [Accessed 15 February 2024].

[144] Montero-Odasso, M. et al., "Gait Velocity as a Single Predictor of Adverse Events in Healthy Seniors Aged 75 Years and Older," *The Journals of Gerontology. Series A: Biological Sciences and Medical Sciences,* vol. 60, no. 10, p. 1304–1309, 2005.

[145] Odonkor, C. A., R. B. Schonberger, F. Dai, K. H. Shelley, D. G. Silverman and P. G. Barash, "New Utility for an Old Tool: Can a Simple Gait Speed Test Predict Ambulatory Surgical Discharge Outcomes?," *American Journal of Physical Medicine and Rehabilitation,* vol. 92, no. 10, p. 849–863, 2013.

[146] Newman, A. B., E. M. Simonsick, B. L. Naydeck, R. M. Boudreau, S. B. Kritchevsky, M. C. Nevitt, M. Pahor, S. Satterfield, J. S. Brach, S. A. Studenski and T. B. Harris, "Association of Long-Distance Corridor Walk Performance With Mortality, Cardiovascular Disease, Mobility Limitation, and Disability," *JAMA,* vol. 295, no. 17, p. 2018–2026, 2006.

[147] Peel, N. M., S. S. Kuys and K. Klein, "Gait Speed as a Measure in Geriatric Assessment in Clinical Settings: a Systematic Review," *The Journals of Gerontology. Series A, Biological Sciences and Medical Sciences,* vol. 68, no. 1, p. 39–46, 2013.

References

[148] Rydwik, E., A. Bergland, L. Forsén and K. Frändin, "Investigation into the Reliability and Validity of the Measurement of Elderly People's Clinical Walking Speed: A Systematic Review," *Physiotherapy Theory and Practice,* vol. 28, no. 3, p. 238–256, 2012.

[149] Alexander, N. B., K. E. Guire, D. G. Thelen, J. A. Ashton-Miller, A. B. Schultz, J. C. Grunawalt and B. Giordani, "Self-Reported Walking Ability Predicts Functional Mobility Performance in Frail Older Adults," *Journal of the American Geriatrics Society,* vol. 48, no. 11, p. 1408–1413, 2000.

[150] Studenski, S. et al., "Physical Performance Measures in the Clinical Setting," *Journal of the American Geriatrics Society,* vol. 51, no. 3, p. 314–322, 2003.

[151] Brach, J. S., S. Perera, J. M. van Swearingen, E. S. Hile, D. M. Wert and S. A. Studenski, "Challenging gait conditions predict 1-year decline in gait speed in older adults with apparently normal gait," *Physical Therapy,* vol. 91, no. 12, p. 1857–1864, 2011.

[152] Artaud, F., A. Singh-Manoux, A. Dugravot, C. Tzourio and A. Elbaz, "Decline in Fast Gait Speed as a Predictor of Disability in Older Adults," *Journal of the American Geriatrics Society,* vol. 63, no. 6, p. 1129–1136, 2015.

[153] Maresova, P. et al., "Activities of Daily Living and Associated Costs in the Most Widespread Neurodegenerative Diseases: A Systematic Review," *Clinical Interventions in Aging,* vol. 15, p. 1841–1862, 2020.

[154] Hobson, P., "Different Stages and Types of Dementia," *Enabling People with Dementia: Understanding and Implementing Person-centred Care,* p. 31–37, 2019.

[155] Dumurgier, J. et al., "Gait Speed and Decline in Gait Speed as Predictors of Incident Dementia," *The Journals of Gerontology. Series A, Biological Sciences and Medical Sciences,* vol. 72, no. 5, p. 655–661, 2017.

[156] Buracchio, T., H. H. Dodge, D. Howieson, D. Wasserman and J. Kaye, "The Trajectory of Gait Speed Preceding Mild Cognitive Impairment," *Archives of Neurology,* vol. 67, no. 8, p. 980–986, 2010.

[157] Kuate-Tegueu, C., J.-A. Avila-Funes, N. Simo, M. le Goff, H. Amiéva, J.-F. Dartigues and M. Tabue-Teguo, "Association of Gait Speed, Psychomotor Speed, and Dementia," *Journal of Alzheimer's Disease,* vol. 60, no. 2, p. 585–592, 2017.

[158] Quan, M. et al., "Walking Pace and the Risk of Cognitive Decline and Dementia in Elderly Populations: A Meta-analysis of Prospective Cohort Studies," *The Journals of Gerontology. Series A, Biological Sciences and Medical Sciences,* vol. 72, no. 2, p. 266–270, 2017.

[159] Morris, R., S. Lord, J. Bunce, D. Burn and L. Rochester, "Gait and Cognition: Mapping the Global and Discrete Relationships in Ageing and Neurodegenerative Disease," *Neuroscience and Biobehavioral Reviews,* vol. 64, p. 326–345, 2016.

[160] Monterro-Odasso, M. et al., "Motor and Cognitive Trajectories Before Dementia: Results from Gait and Brain Study," *Journal of the American Geriatrics Society,* vol. 66, no. 9, p. 1676–1683, 2018.

[161] Hackett, R. A., H. Davies-Kershaw, D. Cadar, M. Orrell and A. Steptoe, "Walking Speed, Cognitive Function, and Dementia Risk in the English Longitudinal Study of Ageing," *Journal of the American Geriatrics Society,* vol. 66, no. 9, p. 1670–1675, 2018.

[162] Mielke, M. et al., "Assessing the Temporal Relationship between Cognition and Gait: Slow Gait Predicts Cognitive Decline in the Mayo Clinic Study of Aging," *The Journals of Gerontology. Series A, Biological Sciences and Medical Sciences,* vol. 68, no. 8, p. 929–937, 2013.

[163] Clouston, S. A. P., P. Brewster, D. Kuh, M. Richards, R. Cooper, R. Hardy, M. S. Rubin and S. M. Hofer, "The Dynamic Relationship between Physical Function and Cognition in Longitudinal Aging Cohorts," *Epidemiologic Reviews,* vol. 35, p. 33–50, 2013.

[164] Blair, C., "How Similar are Fluid Cognition and General Intelligence? A Developmental Neuroscience Perspective on Fluid Cognition as an Aspect of Human Cognitive Ability," *The Behavioral and Brain Sciences,* vol. 29, no. 2, p. 109–125, 2006.

[165] Killane, I., O. A. Donoghue, G. M. Savva, H. Cronin, R. A. Kenny and R. B. Reilly, "Relative Association of Processing Speed, Short-term Memory and Sustained Attention with Task on Gait Speed: A Study of Community-dwelling People 50 Years and Older," *The Journals of Gerontology. Series A, Biological Sciences and Medical Sciences,* vol. 69, no. 11, p. 1407–1411, 2014.

[166] Taniguchi, Y. et al., "Gait Performance Trajectories and Incident Disabling Dementia Among Community-Dwelling Older Japanese," *Journal of the American Medical Directors Association,* vol. 18, no. 2, 2017.

[167] Ben Assayag, E. et al., "Gait Measures as Predictors of Poststroke Cognitive Function: Evidence from the TABASCO Study," *Stroke,* vol. 46, no. 4, p. 1077–1083, 2015.

[168] Hunter, S. W. and A. Divine, "The Effect of Walking Path Configuration on Gait in Adults with Alzheimer's Dementia," *Gait and Posture,* vol. 64, p. 226–229, 2018.

[169] Holtzer, R., C. Wang and J. Verghese, "The Relationship Between Attention and Gait in Aging: Facts and Fallacies," *Motor Control,* vol. 16, no. 1, p. 64–80, 2012.

[170] Welmer, A.-K., D. Rizzuto, C. Qiu, B. Caracciolo and E. J. Laukka, "Walking Speed, Processing Speed, and Dementia: A Population-Based Longitudinal Study," *The Journals of Gerontology. Series A, Biological Sciences and Medical Sciences,* vol. 69, no. 12, p. 1503–1510, 2014.

[171] Tian, Q., E. M. Simonsick, S. M. Resnick, M. D. Shardell, L. Ferrucci and S. A. Studenski, "Lap time Variation and Executive Function in Older Adults: the Baltimore Longitudinal Study of Aging," *Age and Ageing,* vol. 44, no. 5, p. 796–800, 2015.

[172] Tian, Q., S. M. Resnick, L. Ferrucci and S. A. Studenski, "Intra-individual Lap Time Variation of the 400-m Walk, an Early Mobility Indicator of Executive Function Decline in High-Functioning Older Adults?," *Age,* vol. 37, pp. 1-9, 2015.

[173] Mc Ardle, R., R. Morris, J. Wilson, B. Galna, A. J. Thomas and L. Rochester, "What Can Quantitative Gait Analysis Tell Us about Dementia and Its Subtypes? A Structured Review," *Journal of Alzheimer's Disease,* vol. 60, no. 4, p. 1295–1312, 2017.

[174] Ceïde, M. E., E. I. Ayers, R. Lipton and J. Verghese, "Walking While Talking and Risk of Incident Dementia," *The American Journal of Geriatric Psychiatry :*

Official Journal of the American Association for Geriatric Psychiatry, vol. 26, no. 5, p. 580–588, 2018.

[175] Saho, K., K. Uemura, K. Sugano and M. Matsumoto, "Using Micro-Doppler Radar to Measure Gait Features Associated with Cognitive Functions in Elderly Adults," *IEEE Access,* vol. 7, p. 24122–24131, 2019.

[176] Bostan, A. C., R. P. Dum and P. L. Strick, "Cerebellar Networks with the Cerebral Cortex and Basal Ganglia," *Trends in Cognitive Sciences,* vol. 17, no. 5, p. 241–254, 2013.

[177] Eidelberg, E., J. L. Story, J. G. Walden and B. L. Meyer, "Anatomical correlates of return of locomotor function after partial spinal cord lesions in cats," *Experimental Brain Research,* vol. 42, p. 81–88, 1981.

[178] Rosso, A., "Aging, the Central Nervous System, and Mobility," *The Journals of Gerontology. Series A, Biological Sciences and Medical Sciences,* vol. 68, no. 11, p. 1379–1386, 2013.

[179] Callisaya, M. L. et al., "Brain Structural Change and Gait Decline: A Longitudinal Population-Based Study," *Journal of the American Geriatrics Society,* vol. 61, no. 7, p. 1074–1079, 2013.

[180] Srikanth, V. et al., "Cerebral White Matter Lesions, Gait, and the Risk of Incident Falls: a Prospective Population-Based Study," *Stroke,* vol. 40, no. 1, p. 175–180, 2009.

[181] Wennberg, A. M., R. Savica and M. M. Mielke, "Association between Various Brain Pathologies and Gait Disturbance," *Dementia and Geriatric Cognitive Disorders,* vol. 48, no. 3-4, p. 128–143, 2017.

[182] Del Campo, N. et al., "Relationship of Regional Brain β-amyloid to Gait Speed," *Neurology,* vol. 86, no. 1, p. 36–43, 2016.

[183] Brach, J. S., S. Studenski, S. Perera, J. M. van Swearingen and A. B. Newman, "Stance Time and Step Width Variability have Unique Contributing Impairments in Older Persons," *Gait and Posture,* vol. 27, no. 3, p. 431–439, 2008.

[184] Beauchet, O., G. Allali, C. Annweiler and J. Verghese, "Association of Motoric Cognitive Risk Syndrome With Brain Volumes: Results From the GAIT Study," *The Journals of Gerontology. Series A, Biological Sciences and Medical Sciences,* vol. 71, no. 8, p. 1081–1088, 2016.

[185] Allali, G., E. I. Ayers and J. Verghese, "Motoric Cognitive Risk Syndrome Subtypes and Cognitive Profiles," *The Journals of Gerontology. Series A, Biological Sciences and Medical Sciences,* vol. 71, no. 3, p. 378–384, 2016.

[186] Hausdorff, J. M., M. E. Cudkowicz, R. Firtion, J. Y. Wei and A. L. Goldberger, "Gait Variability and Basal Ganglia Disorders: Stride-to-stride Variations of Gait Cycle Timing in Parkinson's Disease and Huntington's Disease," *Movement Disorders : Official Journal of the Movement Disorder Society,* vol. 13, no. 3, p. 428–437, 1998.

[187] Galna, B., S. Lord and L. Rochester, "Is Gait Variability Reliable in Older Adults and Parkinson's Disease? Towards an Optimal Testing Protocol," *Gait and Posture,* vol. 37, no. 4, p. 580–585, 2013.

[188] Frenkel-Toledo, S., N. Giladi, C. Peretz, T. Herman, L. Gruendlinger and J. M. Hausdorff, "Effect of Gait Speed on Gait Rhythmicity in Parkinson's Disease:

Variability of Stride Time and Swing Time Respond Differently," *Journal of Neuroengineering and Rehabilitation*, vol. 2, no. 1, p. 23, 2005.

[189] Amboni, M. et al., "Gait Patterns in Parkinsonian Patients With or Without Mild Cognitive Impairment," *Movement Disorders: Official Journal of the Movement Disorder Society*, vol. 27, no. 12, p. 1536–1543, 2012.

[190] Zeng, W. and C. Wang, "Classification of Neurodegenerative Diseases Using Gait Dynamics via Deterministic Learning," *Information Sciences*, vol. 317, p. 246–258, 2015.

[191] Yan, Y. et al., "Gait Rhythm Dynamics for Neuro-Degenerative Disease Classification via Persistence Landscape- Based Topological Representation," *Sensors*, vol. 20, no. 7, p. 2006, 2020.

[192] Khajuria, A., P. Joshi and D. Joshi, "Comprehensive Statistical Analysis of the Gait Parameters in Neurodegenerative Diseases," *Neurophysiology*, vol. 50, no. 1, p. 38–51, 2018.

[193] Hausdorff, J. et al., "Altered Fractal Dynamics of Gait: Reduced Stride-interval Correlations with Aging and Huntington's Disease," *Journal of Applied Physiology*, vol. 82, no. 1, p. 262–269, 1997.

[194] Callisaya, M. L., L. Blizzard, M. D. Schmidt, K. L. Martin, J. L. McGinley, L. M. Sanders and V. K. Srikanth, "Gait, Gait Variability and the Risk of Multiple Incident Falls in Older People: a Population-based Study," *Age and Ageing*, vol. 40, no. 4, p. 481–487, 2011.

[195] Quach, L. et al., "The Nonlinear Relationship between Gait Speed and Falls: The Maintenance of Balance, Independent Living, Intellect, and Zest in the Elderly of Boston Study," *Journal of the American Geriatrics Society*, vol. 59, no. 6, p. 1069–1073, 2011.

[196] Stone, E., M. Skubic, M. Rantz, C. Abbott and S. Miller, "Average In-home Gait Speed: Investigation of a New Metric for Mobility and Fall Risk Assessment of Elders," *Gait and Posture*, vol. 41, no. 1, p. 57–62, 2015.

[197] Schniepp, R., M. Wuehr, C. Schlick, S. Huth, C. Pradhan, M. Dieterich, T. Brandt and K. Jahn, "Increased Gait Variability is Associated with the History of Falls in Patients with Cerebellar Ataxia," *Journal of Neurology*, vol. 261, no. 1, p. 213–223, 2014.

[198] Dostanpor, A., C. A. Dobson and N. Vanicek, "Relationships between Walking Speed, T-score and Age with Gait Parameters in Plder Post-menopausal Women with Low Bone Mineral Density," *Gait and Posture*, vol. 64, p. 230–237, 2018.

[199] Verghese, J., R. Holtzer, R. B. Lipton and C. Wang, "Quantitative Gait Markers and Incident Fall Risk in Older Adults," *The Journals of Gerontology. Series A, Biological Sciences and Medical Sciences*, vol. 64, no. 8, p. 896–901, 2009.

[200] Hausdorff, J. M., "Gait Variability: Methods, Modeling and Meaning," *Journal of NeuroEngineering and Rehabilitation*, vol. 2, no. 1, pp. 1-9, 2005.

[201] Datta, A., R. Datta and E. J., "What Factors Predict Falls in Older Adults Living in Nursing Homes: A Pilot Study," *Journal of Functional Morphology and Kinesiology 2019*, vol. 4, no. 1, p. 3, 2018.

[202] Reynard, F., P. Vuadens, O. Deriaz and P. Terrier, "Could Local Dynamic Stability Serve as an Early Predictor of Falls in Patients with Moderate Neurological Gait

Disorders? A Reliability and Comparison Study in Healthy Individuals and in Patients with Paresis of the Lower Extremities," *PLoS ONE,* vol. 9, no. 6, p. e100550, 2014.

[203] Toebes, M. J. P., M. J. M. Hoozemans, R. Furrer, J. Dekker and J. H. van Dieën, "Local Dynamic Stability and Variability of Gait are Associated with Fall History in Elderly Subjects," *Gait and Posture,* vol. 36, no. 3, p. 527–531, 2012.

[204] Kasser, S. L., J. V. Jacobs, J. T. Foley, B. J. Cardinal and G. F. Maddalozzo, "A Prospective Evaluation of Balance, Gait, and Strength to Predict Falling in Women with Multiple Sclerosis," *Archives of Physical Medicine and Rehabilitation,* vol. 92, no. 11, p. 1840–1846, 2011.

[205] Saho, K., M. Fujimoto, M. Masugi and L.-S. Chou, "Gait Classification of Young Adults, Elderly Non-Fallers, and Elderly Fallers Using Micro-Doppler Radar Signals: Simulation Study," *IEEE Sensors Journal,* vol. 17, no. 8, p. 2320–2321, 2017.

[206] van Schooten, K. et al., "Ambulatory Fall-Risk Assessment: Amount and Quality of Daily-Life Gait Predict Falls in Older Adults," *The Journals of Gerontology. Series A, Biological Sciences and Medical Sciences,* vol. 70, no. 5, p. 608–615, 2015.

[207] van Schooten, K. S., M. Pijnappels, S. M. Rispens, P. J. M. Elders, P. Lips, A. Daffertshofer, P. J. Beek and J. H. van Dieën, "Daily-Life Gait Quality as Predictor of Falls in Older People: A 1-Year Prospective Cohort Study," *PloS One,* vol. 11, no. 7, p. e0158623, 2016.

[208] White, D. and e. al, "Trajectories of Gait Speed Predict Mortality in Well-Functioning Older Adults: The Health, Aging and Body Composition Study," *The Journals of Gerontology Series A: Biological Sciences and Medical Sciences,* vol. 68, no. 4, pp. 456-464, 2013.

[209] Rosano, C., A. B. Newman, R. Katz, C. H. Hirsch and L. H. Kuller, "Association Between Lower Digit Symbol Substitution Test Score and Slower Gait and Greater Risk of Mortality and of Developing Incident Disability in Well-Functioning Older Adults," *Journal of the American Geriatrics Society,* vol. 56, no. 9, p. 1618–1625, 2008.

[210] Kano, S. et al., "Gait Speed Can Predict Advanced Clinical Outcomes in Patients Who Undergo Transcatheter Aortic Valve Replacement: Insights From a Japanese Multicenter Registry," *Circulation: Cardiovascular Interventions,* vol. 10, no. 9, p. e005088, 2017.

[211] Hecker, F., M. Arsalan, W. Kim and T. Walther, "Transcatheter Aortic Valve Implantation (TAVI) in 2018: Recent Advances and Future Development," *Minerva Cardiology and Angiology,* vol. 66, no. 3, 2018.

[212] Alfredsson, J. et al., "Gait Speed Predicts 30-Day Mortality After Transcatheter Aortic Valve Replacement," *Circulation,* vol. 133, no. 14, p. 1351–1359, 2016.

[213] Afilalo, J. et al., "Gait Speed as an Incremental Predictor of Mortality and Major Morbidity in Elderly Patients Undergoing Cardiac Surgery," *Journal of the American College of Cardiology,* vol. 56, no. 20, p. 1668–1676, 2010.

[214] Stamatakis, E. et al., "Self-Rated Walking Pace and All-Cause, Cardiovascular Disease and Cancer Mortality: Individual Participant Pooled Analysis of 50 225

Walkers from 11 Population British Cohorts," *British Journal of Sports Medicine,* vol. 52, no. 12, pp. 761-768, 2018.

[215] Afilalo, J. et al., "Gait Speed and 1-Year Mortality Following Cardiac Surgery: A Landmark Analysis From the Society of Thoracic Surgeons Adult Cardiac Surgery Database," *Journal of the American Heart Association,* vol. 7, no. 23, p. e010139, 2018.

[216] Studenski, S., "Gait Speed and Survival in Older Adults," *JAMA,* vol. 305, no. 1, p. 50, 2011.

[217] Hardy, S. E., S. Perera, Y. F. Roumani, J. M. Chandler and S. A. Studenski, "Improvement in Usual Gait Speed Predicts Better Survival in Older Adults," *Journal of the American Geriatrics Society,* vol. 55, no. 11, p. 1727–1734, 2007.

[218] Ayers, E. and J. Verghese, "Motoric Cognitive Risk Syndrome and Risk of Mortality in Older Adults," *Alzheimer's and Dementia,* vol. 12, no. 5, p. 556–564, 2016.

[219] Kutner, N. G., R. Zhang, Y. Huang and P. Painter, "Gait Speed and Mortality, Hospitalization, and Functional Status Change Among Hemodialysis Patients: A US Renal Data System Special Study," *American Journal of Kidney Diseases,* vol. 66, no. 2, p. 297–304, 2015.

[220] Welmer, A.-K., S. Angleman, E. Rydwik, L. Fratiglioni and C. Qiu, "Association of Cardiovascular Burden with Mobility Limitation among Elderly People: A Population-Based Study," *PLoS ONE,* vol. 8, no. 5, p. e65815, 2013.

[221] Heiland, E. G., C. Qiu, R. Wang, G. Santoni, Y. Liang, L. Fratiglioni and A.-K. Welmer, "Cardiovascular Risk Burden and Future Risk of Walking Speed Limitation in Older Adults," *Journal of the American Geriatrics Society,* vol. 65, no. 11, p. 2418–2424, 2017.

[222] Jin, Y., T. Tanaka, Y. Ma, S. Bandinelli, L. Ferrucci and S. A. Talegawkar, "Cardiovascular Health Is Associated With Physical Function Among Older Community Dwelling Men and Women," *The Journals of Gerontology: Series A,* vol. 72, no. 12, p. 1710–1716, 2017.

[223] McGinn, A. et al., "Walking Speed and Risk of Incident Ischemic Stroke Among Postmenopausal Women," *Stroke,* vol. 39, no. 4, p. 1233–1239, 2008.

[224] Zeki Al Hazzouri, A. et al., "Perceived Walking Speed, Measured Tandem Walk, Incident Stroke, and Mortality in Older Latino Adults: A Prospective Cohort Study," *The Journals of Gerontology Series A: Biological Sciences and Medical Sciences,* vol. 72, no. 5, pp. 676-682, 2016.

[225] van de Port, I., G. Kwakkel and E. Lindeman, "Community Ambulation in Patients with Chronic Stroke: How is it Related to Gait Speed?," *Journal of Rehabilitation Medicine,* vol. 40, no. 1, p. 23–27, 2008.

[226] Altenburger, P. et al., "Examination of Sustained Gait Speed During Extended Walking in Individuals With Chronic Stroke," *Archives of Physical Medicine and Rehabilitation,* vol. 941, no. 12, p. 2471–2477, 2013.

[227] An, S., Y. Lee, H. Shin and G. Lee, "Gait Velocity and Walking Distance to Predict Community Walking after Stroke," *Nursing and Health Sciences,* vol. 17, no. 4, p. 533–538, 2015.

[228] Margolis, R. and A. M. Verdery, "Older Adults Without Close Kin in the United States," *The Journals of Gerontology: Series B,* vol. 72, no. 4, p. 688–693, 2017.
[229] Sanders, J. B., M. A. Bremmer, D. J. H. Deeg and A. T. F. Beekman, "Do Depressive Symptoms and Gait Speed Impairment Predict Each Other's Incidence? A 16-Year Prospective Study in the Community," *Journal of the American Geriatrics Society,* vol. 60, no. 9, p. 1673–1680, 2012.
[230] Selge, C., F. Schoeberl, A. Zwergal, G. Nuebling, T. Brandt, M. Dieterich, R. Schniepp and K. Jahn, "Gait Analysis in PSP and NPH," *Neurology,* vol. 90, no. 12, p. e1021–e1028, 2018.

Index

A

acute, 1, 6, 46, 50, 55, 78
advancement(s), xi, 1, 39, 71, 94
aging-related, 1
anterior-posterior, 4, 48
application(s), xi, 1, 2, 21, 24, 25, 27, 38, 94, 97, 99, 100, 102, 104, 105
artificial intelligence-driven, xi, 94

B

biomechanics, 1, 99, 103, 105
biomedical engineers, 1

C

cardiovascular, vii, xi, 1, 9, 45, 46, 47, 49, 64, 79, 81, 82, 83, 84, 85, 91, 93, 97, 106, 111, 112
cardiovascular risk, vii, 82, 83, 84, 85, 112
central nervous system, vii, 62, 63, 64, 67, 68, 69, 73, 91, 109
clinicians, xi, 1, 12, 46, 47, 51
cognition, 1, 6, 31, 52, 54, 55, 58, 59, 62, 71, 93, 97, 107, 108
contact devices, vii, 11, 28, 39
continuous wave (CW), 20, 21, 26, 100, 101

D

decline of cognitive function, vii, 51, 58
dementia, vii, 1, 51, 52, 53, 54, 55, 56, 57, 58, 59, 60, 61, 65, 91, 92, 93, 95, 97, 107, 108, 109, 112
detection, 1, 12, 20, 21, 29, 38, 51, 91, 94, 102
disease(s), xi, 1, 4, 5, 7, 9, 20, 31, 45, 46, 48, 49, 51, 53, 55, 57, 59, 60, 61, 64, 65, 66, 67, 68, 69, 78, 79, 81, 82, 83, 84, 91, 92, 93, 94, 95, 97, 98, 103, 104, 106, 107, 108, 109, 110, 111, 112

E

electromyography (EMG), 3, 14

F

fall prediction, vii, 70, 71, 74, 77, 91
foot, 1, 3, 4, 5, 12, 17, 20, 25, 28, 29, 30, 33, 37, 39, 40, 46, 72, 82, 103, 104, 105, 106
footwear and insoles, 39
force plates, 11, 17, 18, 100
frailty, 1, 19, 97

G

gait analysis, vii, xi, 1, 3, 6, 9, 11, 12, 13, 14, 15, 17, 18, 19, 23, 25, 28, 29, 31, 34, 35, 36, 37, 38, 39, 41, 42, 51, 58, 60, 62, 65, 67, 70, 73, 74, 77, 80, 82, 84, 85, 87, 88, 91, 92, 94, 96, 97, 98, 99, 100, 101, 102, 103, 105, 106, 108, 113
gait assessment, xi, 1, 3, 6, 12, 13, 94

H

healthcare, xi, 94, 96, 100

Index

I

impairment(s), 1, 51, 52, 53, 58, 64, 65, 66, 67, 69, 71, 73, 78, 82, 88, 94, 104, 107, 109, 110, 113
infrared thermal cameras, 11, 18

L

long-term, 1, 32, 54

M

mobility, 1, 7, 31, 36, 46, 47, 48, 49, 51, 59, 63, 68, 70, 76, 83, 84, 94, 96, 97, 98, 103, 106, 107, 108, 109, 110, 112
monitoring, 1, 2, 28, 36, 45, 51, 70, 76, 77, 79, 83, 85, 88, 94, 96, 101, 102, 103, 104
monograph, xi, 1, 2, 9, 11, 94, 96
mortality, vii, 46, 49, 77, 78, 79, 80, 81, 82, 83, 87, 91, 93, 95, 106, 111, 112
motion, xi, 1, 4, 7, 9, 11, 15, 17, 20, 21, 24, 25, 26, 29, 30, 37, 40, 41, 43, 48, 50, 66, 67, 71, 73, 76, 92, 94, 95, 99, 100, 101, 103, 105, 106
motion capture, xi, 1, 4, 7, 11, 15, 21, 30, 43, 48, 50, 66, 67, 71, 73, 76, 92, 95, 99, 101
movement(s), xi, xii, 1, 13, 15, 20, 21, 24, 25, 31, 37, 48, 51, 62, 63, 73, 94, 96, 100, 104, 105, 109, 110

N

neurological pathology, 1, 88
neurology, xi, 1, 63, 97, 103, 107, 109, 110, 113
non-contact devices, 11

O

older adults, 1, 4, 7, 8, 13, 17, 29, 30, 34, 36, 46, 48, 49, 50, 57, 59, 67, 68, 70, 73, 74, 75, 76, 77, 79, 80, 84, 94, 107

P

parameters, vii, ix, 1, 3, 4, 5, 6, 7, 8, 9, 11, 12, 13, 15, 17, 18, 20, 21, 22, 23, 24, 26, 27, 29, 31, 33, 34, 35, 36, 37, 39, 40, 41, 42, 47, 48, 49, 51, 54, 55, 57, 59, 61, 63, 64, 65, 66, 67, 68, 69, 71, 72, 73, 75, 76, 77, 86, 87, 91, 92, 93, 94, 95, 97, 98, 99, 100, 101, 103, 104, 105, 110
pathological, xi, 33, 45
physical, 1, 3, 6, 11, 17, 23, 29, 30, 38, 49, 58, 70, 77, 84, 85, 98, 99, 103, 104, 105, 106, 107, 108, 111, 112
prediction, 57, 86, 87, 91, 95
pressure mats and walkways, 11

R

radar systems, vii, 19, 20, 21, 26
rehabilitation, xi, 1, 33, 37, 38, 40, 86, 94, 98, 103, 104, 105, 106, 110, 111, 112

S

scientific, xi
sensors, 11, 12, 13, 14, 18, 19, 21, 23, 24, 28, 29, 30, 31, 32, 34, 35, 36, 37, 39, 40, 42, 56, 58, 65, 69, 71, 73, 74, 77, 92, 95, 97, 99, 100, 101, 102, 103, 104, 105, 110, 111
spatiotemporal, vii, 3, 5, 6, 8, 13, 17, 18, 20, 23, 29, 31, 33, 34, 36, 40, 41, 98, 99, 100, 104, 105, 106
speed, vii, 3, 4, 5, 6, 7, 8, 9, 12, 14, 15, 17, 18, 19, 22, 24, 25, 27, 28, 29, 32, 34, 36, 37, 38, 40, 41, 42, 43, 45, 46, 47, 48, 49, 50, 52, 53, 54, 55, 56, 57, 58, 59, 60, 61, 62, 63, 64, 66, 67, 68, 69, 70, 71, 72, 74, 75, 76, 77, 78, 79, 80, 81, 82, 83, 84, 85, 86, 87, 88, 91, 92, 93, 94, 97, 98, 99, 100, 101, 102, 106, 107, 108, 109, 110, 111, 112, 113
step-to-step, 5
stride analyzers, 42, 43
stroke, vii, 9, 41, 55, 61, 78, 85, 86, 87, 91, 92, 93, 95, 106, 108, 109, 112

T

technique(s), xi, 20
timed up-and-go (TUG), 6, 7, 9, 55, 70

W

walking, xi, 1, 3, 4, 5, 6, 7, 8, 9, 12, 13, 15, 17, 18, 19, 21, 22, 23, 24, 25, 26, 27, 28, 30, 31, 33, 34, 36, 37, 38, 39, 40, 42, 45, 46, 47, 48, 49, 50, 52, 53, 54, 55, 56, 57, 58, 59, 60, 61, 62, 63, 66, 69, 70, 71, 72, 73, 74, 75, 76, 77, 79, 81, 83, 84, 85, 86, 87, 88, 92, 97, 98, 99, 101, 102, 103, 104, 105, 107, 108, 110, 111, 112

wearable sensors, xi, 1, 29, 39
wearables and inertial measurements units (IMU), 23, 28, 29, 30, 32, 34, 35, 36, 37, 38, 39, 40, 103, 105, 106